Chatham House Report

Charles Clift
May 2014

What's the World Health Organization For?

Final Report from the Centre on Global Health Security Working Group on Health Governance

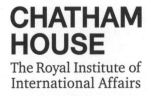

CHATHAM HOUSE
The Royal Institute of
International Affairs

Chatham House has been the home of the Royal Institute of International Affairs for more than ninety years. Our mission is to be a world-leading source of independent analysis, informed debate and influential ideas on how to build a prosperous and secure world for all.

The Royal Institute of International Affairs

Chatham House
10 St James's Square
London SW1Y 4LE
T: +44 (0) 20 7957 5700
F: + 44 (0) 20 7957 5710
www.chathamhouse.org

Charity Registration No. 208223

ISBN 978 1 78413 020 6

A catalogue record for this title is available from the British Library.

Cover image © WHO/Pierre Albouy

Typeset by Soapbox, www.soapbox.co.uk

Printed by Latimer Trend and Co Ltd

FSC

Contents

About the Author

Charles Clift is a Senior Consulting Fellow in the Centre on Global Health Security at Chatham House. Previously he was an economist at the UK Department for International Development. In addition to his work for Chatham House, Dr Clift has been a consultant to UNITAID, the World Intellectual Property Organization, the Access to Medicine Foundation and the World Health Organization, where he was a staff member from 2004 to 2006.

Acronyms and Abbreviations

AFRO	WHO Regional Office for Africa	JIU	Joint Inspection Unit
A&M	Administrative and management	MDG(s)	Millennium Development Goal(s)
AMRO	WHO Regional Office for the Americas	MMV	Medicines for Malaria Venture
ASEAN	Association of Southeast Asian Nations	OAS	Organization of American States
AU	African Union	PAHO	Pan American Health Organization
DNDi	Drugs for Neglected Diseases initiative	PASB	Pan American Sanitary Bureau
EB	Executive Board	PASO	Pan American Sanitary Organization
EMRO	WHO Regional Office for the Eastern Mediterranean	PEPFAR	US President's Emergency Plan for AIDS Relief
EURO	WHO Regional Office for Europe	RD	Regional Director
FCTC	Framework Convention on Tobacco Control	SEARO	WHO Regional Office for South-East Asia
Global Fund	Global Fund to Fight AIDS, Tuberculosis and Malaria	UNCERF	UN Central Emergency Response Fund
		WHA	World Health Assembly
GPG	Global Policy Group	WHO	World Health Organization
GPW	General Programme of Work	WPRO	WHO Regional Office for the Western Pacific
IHME	Institute of Health Metrics and Evaluation		
IHR	International Health Regulations	WR	WHO Representative

'I thought I knew WHO very well, but when I became the Regional Director I felt overwhelmed. The Organization has such a complexity. Personally, I have substantial experience in managing organizations but this organization is the most complex. I think it may be one of the most complex organizations that exists.'

Dr Shin Young-soo, WHO Regional Director for the Western Pacific (Interview with Dr Anne Marie Worning, March 2014, http://www.who.int/about/who_reform/matrix-management/en/.)

Preface

The Chatham House Working Group on Health Governance was formed to consider, in the first instance, the role of the World Health Organization (WHO) in the international system that supports global health. This was done in the knowledge that the WHO had recently embarked on a programme of reform, which had its roots in the acute funding pressures that it was experiencing. It was therefore envisaged as a complementary exercise to the internal reform process. The WHO's Director-General, Margaret Chan, welcomed the initiative, saying:

> We are happy to hear different views and suggestions on the WHO reform. There are many reasons why WHO should embrace change to be relevant and responsive to global health challenges. The complex mechanism of financing in WHO is a major problem that needs to be addressed […] as some Geneva-based Ambassadors used to say 'the current financing of WHO is a barrier to the Organization's effectiveness'.

The perceived advantage of an outside body (some members of which are also active participants in the internal reform process) is the ability to step outside the constraints that are inevitable in the formal processes of an intergovernmental body, and to consider issues that are important but politically difficult to address.

The members of the group met three times: in October 2012 at Chatham House; in April 2013 in Bangkok; and, for the last time, in October 2013 at Chatham House. The names of members and others involved from time to time are in Annex 1. Three background papers were commissioned and published.[1] In addition, numerous short internal papers were produced to aid the group's discussions. The group benefited from the feedback from the members of the companion working group on health financing.

Most members of the group wanted to find a way to strengthen the WHO in order that it should play its proper role as a leader in the global health arena. They did not support the view that the WHO has been rendered largely redundant as a result of the proliferation of other national and international institutions with a role in promoting global health; rather the opposite. Now that the infrastructure of global health had become infinitely more complex than it was when the WHO was founded in 1948, an effective WHO was more important than ever. A revitalized WHO was equally important in order to address the new health challenges now confronting the world, not least that of tackling non-communicable diseases.

The WHO's unique strengths were recognized. Its advice is still respected globally because it can draw on the best brains in the world to provide their expertise to the WHO. It has an unparalleled extensive worldwide network – not just its own offices, but also its collaborating centres. It has a convening power greater than that of any other global health institution. The global brand of 'WHO' remains uniquely powerful.

Others in the group were more sceptical about the ability of the WHO (and its member states) to bring about reform (or indeed that of the wider UN to do so) and therefore favoured various initiatives that would involve hiving off some WHO functions to other bodies or other forums. Such ideas are discussed at various points in this report.

The group had lively and productive discussions throughout. Many different perspectives and ideas were proposed and subjected to scrutiny. There was consensus in a number of areas on the role that the WHO should ideally play, but less agreement concerning what kind of restructuring might or might not be desirable or possible to help the WHO play that role. Accordingly, this report seeks to present the arguments made for reform of the WHO, the various ways this could be done and the obstacles to implementing these reforms. It seeks to reflect accurately the different shades of opinion expressed within the group.

It is therefore a work of discussion and analysis based on the deliberations of the group, but any views expressed are those of the author, not the responsibility of the group, or indeed of Chatham House.

Finally, thanks are due for the generous support of our funders: the Bill & Melinda Gates Foundation, the UK Department for International Development, the Rockefeller Foundation and the Skoll Foundation. They also bear no responsibility for any views expressed.

Charles Clift
Chatham House
May 2014

---

[1] Clift, C., 'The Role of the World Health Organization in the International System', Working Group Paper, February 2013; Lidén, J. 'The Grand Decade for Global Health: 1998–2008', Working Group Paper, April 2013; Nambiar D. et al., 'The World Health Organization in the South East Asia Region: Decision-maker Perceptions', Working Paper, April 2014. Available at: http://www.chathamhouse.org/research/global-health-security/current-projects/identifying-sustainable-methods-improving-global-he.

Executive Summary and Recommendations

The Chatham House Working Group on Health Governance, in the institute's Centre on Global Health Security, was formed to consider, in the first instance, the role of the World Health Organization (WHO) in the international system that supports global health.

The members of the group met three times. There was broad consensus on the role that the WHO should ideally play, but views differed concerning what kind of restructuring might or might not be desirable or possible to help it play that role. This report is intended as a complementary contribution to the ongoing internal debate on the reform of the WHO, but offers a perspective based on the deliberations of a group that was able to step outside the constraints inevitable in the formal processes of an intergovernmental body, and to consider issues that are important but politically difficult to address. While this report is based on the deliberations of the group, any views expressed are those of the author, not the responsibility of the group, or indeed of Chatham House.

A changed world

Much has changed in the world since the WHO was founded in 1948 – politically and economically, as well as in global health. The Iron Curtain has come and gone. The world's economy and technical capacity have expanded beyond what anyone then could have imagined. The Western economies have experienced unprecedented growth, but their economic and political dominance is now being challenged by the rapidly growing economies of countries emerging from developing status. As a result, there is accompanying uncertainty about how global institutions, which reflect the post-war status quo, can adapt to a world so different.

At the same time, the health status of most people in most countries has improved as a result of better resourcing of health services, technology development and improvement in living conditions arising from economic growth and the accompanying greater capacity to invest in social determinants of health such as education, and water and sanitation. However, although progress has been made, it has not been sufficient for the most part to meet the targets set in the Millennium Development Goals – for example reducing the under-5 mortality rate by two-thirds and the maternal mortality ratio by three-quarters between 1990 and 2015.

Beyond this, the global health community – including the WHO – has struggled to address threats to global health and security, ranging from climate change, population growth and environmental degradation to the spread of communicable and non-communicable disease, migration, and rising inequalities associated with globalization and the failure sufficiently to improve many of the social determinants of health. These threats often emerge initially in other sectors and involve issues with which health professionals are unfamiliar and which they are powerless to influence.

There has been a proliferation of new global health institutions, driven in particular by the rapid increase in development assistance for health that occurred in the first decade of the century. Notable among these are the Global Fund to Fight AIDS, Tuberculosis and Malaria, the GAVI Alliance, UNITAID and public–private partnerships for product development. These new institutions have also pioneered new forms of governance by including alongside governments representatives of civil society, the private sector and foundations.

Meanwhile, the WHO has launched a comprehensive internal reform programme, driven by a potential funding crisis related to stagnation in funding after a long period of growth, as well as excessive reliance on uncertain and inflexible funding from voluntary contributions and grants which made realistic planning and effective management difficult.

But within this reform programme, there are key issues that are not really discussed because – although of great importance – they are politically difficult to deal with. External commentators, including some who have previously worked for the WHO, complain that it is too politicized, too bureaucratic, too dominated by medical staff seeking medical solutions to what are often social and economic problems, too timid in approaching controversial issues, too overstretched and too slow to adapt to change.

In particular, numerous external reports going back more than 20 years have identified key problems arising from the WHO's unique configuration of six regional offices, with directors elected by member states, and its extensive network of about 150 country offices. While these reports have recommended sometimes radical reforms, there has been hardly any response from the WHO and its member states. This is because the governance structures in the WHO mean that there is a very strong interest in maintaining the status quo. It is also the case that those relatively few member states that provide the majority of funding for the WHO have hitherto never felt it sufficiently important to devote the time and effort required to bring about reforms that would inevitably be contentious and disruptive in the short term.

The working group challenged the mythology of a 'golden age' in which the WHO actually performed the function of being the directing and coordinating body in international health. According to this mythology, the history of the WHO has been one of a downward slide during which it has gradually lost its erstwhile authority, which has passed to the multitude of other global health agencies. In this view, the very existence of organizations such as GAVI or the Global Fund is a reminder of the WHO's failure, and of the extent to which the international community (particularly the donor community) prefers to bypass a WHO that is perceived as clodhopping and ineffective.

However, the working group was very clear that the WHO had never been intended as a body that should undertake each and every function which might contribute to global health. It was not intended to be a funding agency, or indeed a research organization. Moreover, the new and more complex institutional structure in global health that accompanied the increase in funding was also to be welcomed. While there were drawbacks to this proliferation of funding bodies, the new infrastructure also offered more choice for countries seeking funding or technical assistance and innovation in governance structures, as well as in funding methods. An element of competition to traditional providers such as the World Bank and the WHO was, on balance, considered a good thing.

The current programme of reform is an opportunity for the WHO and its member states to think more fundamentally about the organization's role in this changed global environment. The proliferation of global health institutions, perceived by some as a threat, is in fact an opportunity for the WHO to define better a much-needed coordinating role in this far more complex institutional environment. The WHO also has an important role to play in influencing other actors within and outside the health sector – both governmental and non-governmental – to behave in ways that seek to reconcile the political, economic and commercial objectives of these actors with public health goals.

What should the WHO do?

Recommendation 1: The WHO's core functions should explicitly provide for its work in promoting and maintaining global health security.

The WHO has a dual role as a provider of global public goods that benefit all nations – rich and poor – and that need to be provided collectively, and as a provider of supportive services to its member states. The WHO's current definition of its core functions provides a sound basis for the future, but given their level of generality these may not capture explicitly certain functions that are important, or may implicitly include functions that are less important. For example, there is no specific mention of a role in relation to ensuring global health security such as the WHO's role in global health security, which involves, for instance, action around international public health emergencies and pandemics.

Recommendation 2: The WHO should provide strategic technical assistance to countries in support of its mission as a provider of global public goods. It should not seek to undertake activities that could or should be done better by others – by the host government, with or without support from other agencies.

The nature of the WHO's leadership role is largely undefined in the current core functions. This is with regard to both the health sector and relationships with governmental and non-governmental actors, and regarding decisions and actions outside the health sector that have an impact on health. Nor do the current core functions adequately describe what sort of technical assistance the WHO should be offering to member countries. Technical assistance offered to members should be related to the WHO's core remit of providing normative, standard-setting and other services – broadly the provision of global public goods for health.

Recommendation 3: The WHO should undertake a review of the skills mix and expertise of its staff to ensure that these fit with its core functions and leadership priorities.

The WHO's professional staff are predominantly either health professionals or administrators. Addressing the social, economic and environmental determinants of health and non-communicable disease, and advising countries on the attainment of universal health coverage and financial protection would seem to demand a very different distribution of skills from that which exists currently. Because the WHO has a rapid turnover of staff, significant changes could be made in a relatively short period of time.

Governance of the WHO: the global role

Recommendation 4: The WHO should provide an internal separation between its technical departments and those dealing with governance and management by creating two posts of deputy director-general, with one to be responsible for each.

The WHO is both a technical agency and a policy-making body. The excessive intrusion of political considerations in its technical work can damage its authority and credibility as a standard-bearer for health. Determined leadership is necessary to overcome political and economic interests that threaten public health goals. But politics cannot realistically be wholly separated from the WHO's technical work. However, this is one proposal that may reduce the harmful effects of politicization.

Recommendation 5: The WHO should allow the director-general a single, seven-year term, without the possibility of re-election.

Having previously had no limit on the number of five-year terms that the director-general and regional directors could serve, in the 1990s the WHO introduced a limit of two terms (i.e. renewable once) for these posts. This was partly in response to concerns about the harmful impact of electoral considerations on the governance of the organization. This could be carried further and is a second proposal that may reduce the harmful effects of politicization.

Recommendation 6: The WHO should explore new avenues for collaboration with non-governmental actors that have a concrete and specific purpose.

The WHO's plans for greater involvement of non-governmental stakeholders in its processes seem to have reached a dead end. This is for a number of reasons, including concerns of some member states about diluting the sovereignty of governments in the WHO, the difficulty of managing conflicts of interest, and lack of agreement and trust between stakeholders. It is also because the proposals to date for greater involvement have no concrete goals beyond the desire to involve stakeholders, as important players in the health sector, in the WHO's deliberative processes. It was observed that collaboration with these stakeholders has been most successful where it is built around tackling more specific tasks or problems where mutual confidence and trust can be built through constructive endeavour.

Governance of the WHO: regions and countries

Recommendation 7: The WHO should consider two alternative proposals for restructuring its regional offices:

- *Unitary*: The WHO should be like other UN organizations, where the need for regional (and country) offices is determined by what makes sense in terms of achieving organizational objectives. Elected regional directors should be phased out in order to allow structural changes to take place.

- *Decentralized*: The WHO should apply the Pan American Health Organization (PAHO) model to the other regional offices; and the assessed contribution should be provided to regional offices directly by regional member states, rather than redistributed by headquarters in Geneva. This would involve accepting a decentralized model in the WHO – or even the complete autonomy of regional offices, or their absorption by other regional organizations.

The WHO's unique regional structure is deeply embedded in history and in its political dynamics. While there is a widespread recognition that its decentralized structure entails significant costs and inefficiencies, which are manifested in different ways, there is also a pervasive resignation about the possibility of effecting any significant change in the current model. Most members of the working group supported changes in principle. They discussed, but did not agree on, these two alternative proposals.

Recommendation 8: A comprehensive and independent review – of the kind that has been suggested since 1997 – is overdue to examine how the staffing of country offices should be matched to the needs of host countries, in particular with a view to translating WHO recommendations into practice.

The essential purpose and staffing of country offices, the activities and skill sets required, and how they should be distributed in the light of varying and evolving country needs have long been debated within the WHO. But, like the regional offices, and for many of the same reasons, there have always been grounds for not pursuing these issues with any vigour. The reform programme is an opportunity to do this.

Financing of the WHO

Recommendation 9: The WHO and its member states should examine how its effectiveness could be enhanced by reviewing – in conjunction with the other recommendations in this report – how the value added by its regional and country offices could be increased, and its administrative and management costs reduced.

The WHO has been reliant on voluntary contributions even from its early days, but in the last five years the share of these in funding has exceeded 75 per cent. The WHO's problem is not inadequate income. Rather, it is the imbalance between what member states, through the governing bodies, and voluntary contributors (including member states), through separate agreements, ask the WHO to do. Any programme of reform needs to undertake a serious review of the major cost centres – in particular administration and management, the cost of which is directly related to the WHO's extensive network of country and regional offices, and to the governance mechanisms associated with its unique regional structure. This needs to be done in the context of considering what functions the WHO should be undertaking, and what can be done at least as well by others. This report argues that a comprehensive reform programme should concentrate on these structural issues concerning governance and cost-effectiveness, and that a WHO focused on its core tasks could do more good with less money. The WHO's member states have so far been unwilling to tackle these structural issues in the reform programme.

1. A Changed World

Introduction

The World Health Organization (WHO) was founded in 1948, in the immediate aftermath of the Second World War, with the idealism and ambition that marked the creation of the United Nations system as a whole. The idealism was apparent in its objective – 'the attainment by all peoples of the highest possible level of health' – and the ambition in the 22 wide-ranging functions defined in its constitution, of which the first was 'to act as the directing and co-ordinating authority on international health work'.

Much has changed since 1948 in the world at large, and in that of global health. The Second World War is now part of history, rather than the all-pervading nightmare from which the world was struggling to escape when the WHO was founded. The global economy and technical capacity have expanded beyond what anyone then could have imagined. The political landscape has also been transformed. The Iron Curtain has come and gone. The Western economies have experienced unprecedented growth – now faltering – and their economic and political dominance is now challenged by the rapidly growing economies of countries emerging from developing status. As a result, there is accompanying uncertainty about how global institutions, reflecting the post-war status quo, can adapt to a world so different. The dramatic shifts in global economic status since 1990 are well captured in Figure 1.

Figure 1: Changes in country economic status, 1990–2011

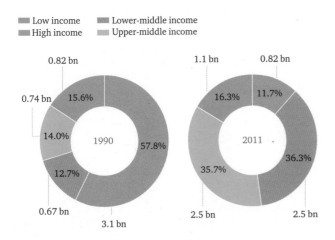

- Low income
- Lower-middle income
- High income
- Upper-middle income

Source: Lancet Commission on Investing in Health.

Beyond this, the world – including the global health community – has struggled with how to address the perceived threats to global health and security, ranging from climate change, population growth and environmental degradation to the spread of communicable and non-communicable disease, migration, and rising inequalities associated with globalization and the failure sufficiently to improve many of the social determinants of health. These threats often emerge in other sectors and involve issues with which health professionals are unfamiliar and that they are powerless to influence.

Better health

Much has also changed in the state of global health, while much has remained unaltered. There has undoubtedly been progress. Since the Millennium Development Goals (MDGs) were established in 2000, the world has made some astonishing strides towards better health, although not all the MDG health-related targets will be achieved.

One of our background papers described the period 1998–2008 as the 'Grand Decade for Global Health'.[2] The 2013 Lancet Commission on Investing in Health[3] noted the impressive reductions in mortality in low- and middle-income countries achieved in the 20 years since the publication of the World Bank's 1993 *World Development Report on Investing in Health*.[4] The commission attributed this improvement to the better technologies that have become available as a result of investment in research and development, and to the transformation in the 'financing, architecture and governance of global health […] in ways that were scarcely imaginable two decades ago'. On the other hand, the Lancet report underplayed the importance of the economic and social improvements that have contributed to these health gains, and the importance of addressing these determinants of health in the future if such gains are to continue.[5]

These health improvements include the following:

- Between 1990 and 2012 the under-five mortality rate declined by 47 per cent; and the average annual rate of decline in the last seven years has been more than triple that in 1900–95. An impressive achievement, but insufficient to reach the MDG target of a reduction by two-thirds in the child mortality rate between 1990 and 2015.

[2] Lidén, J., 'The Grand Decade for Global Health: 1998–2008', April 2013, http://www.chathamhouse.org/sites/default/files/public/Research/Global%20Health/0413_who.pdf.

[3] Jamison, D. et al., 'Global Health 2035: A World Converging within a Generation', *The Lancet*, Vol. 382, 7 December 2013, http://globalhealth2035.org/sites/default/files/report/global-health-2035.pdf.

[4] World Bank, *World Development Report,* Washington DC, 1993, http://files.dcp2.org/pdf/WorldDevelopmentReport1993.pdf.

[5] Clift, C., 'Global Health 2035: The 1993 World Development Report Revisited', Chatham House, 2013, http://www.chathamhouse.org/media/comment/view/195864.

- The maternal mortality ratio nearly halved between 1990 and 2010, but this was insufficient to get near to the MDG target of a reduction by three-quarters.

- Malaria deaths fell by 26 per cent between 2000 and 2010; and mortality due to tuberculosis has fallen by 45 per cent since 1990.

- The number of people newly infected with HIV fell from 3.4 million in 2001 to 2.3 million in 2012; and the number of deaths fell from a peak of 2.3 million in 2005 to 1.6 million in 2012.

New challenges

The WHO's historical concentration has been, and continues to be, on tackling infectious diseases.[6] One aspect of the successes in tackling infectious diseases and child mortality is that non-communicable diseases are now the principal cause of illness and premature death in most parts of the world. The international community and the WHO are only now coming to grips with the implications of these profound changes in the global burden of disease. These will require major changes in the WHO's approach, including addressing those practices of industries such as food and beverages that may contribute to the problem.[7] The WHO's major achievement to date in this field has been the Framework Convention on Tobacco Control (FCTC), but in spite of this the number of smokers globally continues to rise.[8] There is a large agenda that the WHO has begun to map out with its recently approved Global Action Plan for the Prevention and Control of Noncommunicable Diseases 2013–2020.[9]

Regarding country needs for support from the WHO, another fundamental change has been the development of indigenous capacity in the field of health, which profoundly alters the nature of the support and advice that countries may need and expect from the WHO. Militating against this development of national capacity has been the massive rise in the international migration of health workers as a result of increased ability to train health workers and the economic opportunities that globalization has opened up for them. The WHO has to date responded more to the latter trend by drawing up its Global Code of Practice on the International Recruitment of Health Personnel.[10]

However, the WHO has not comprehensively reviewed the nature of the support that it provides to countries. As early as 1997 a special group established to look at its constitution concluded that the WHO should provide advice and technical cooperation to countries on ways to strengthen and improve sustainable health systems and resources, and on enhancing policy-making, management capability and accountability within their health systems.[11] But little has been done to reorient how the WHO works with countries.

Although the importance of other economic and social sectors to health status is partly reflected in the WHO constitution, the issue of how the WHO – as an agency staffed principally by health professionals – should address the health implications of actions in other sectors is a perennial source of unresolved debate. This agenda was prominent in the declaration of the Alma-Ata conference in 1978,[12] which reinforced the WHO's 'Health for All' policy, in the Ottawa Charter for Health Promotion of 1986[13] and in subsequent health promotion conferences that have latterly adopted 'Health in All Policies' to represent the need for inter-sectoral action to promote health.[14] The follow-up to the 2008 Commission on the Social Determinants of Health imposed an obligation to increase its capacity to promote addressing social determinants of health in order to reduce health inequities as an objective across all the WHO's work.[15] Nevertheless, the WHO has not committed any substantial resources to this task. Similarly, new environmental concerns such as climate change have further added to the range of duties that member states expect the WHO to undertake.[16] The impact of intellectual property rights on pharmaceutical innovation and access to medicines has been the subject of intense but unresolved negotiations in the WHO for more

---

[6] Stuckler, D. et al., 'WHO's Budgetary Allocations and Burden of Disease: A Comparative Analysis', *The Lancet*, Vol. 372 (9649):1563–69.

[7] Resolution A66.2. Political Declaration of the High-level Meeting of the General Assembly on the Prevention and Control of Non-communicable Diseases, September 2011, http://www.who.int/nmh/events/un_ncd_summit2011/political_declaration_en.pdf.

[8] Ng, Marie et al., 'Smoking Prevalence and Cigarette Consumption in 187 Countries, 1980–2012', *JAMA* (2014), 311(2):183–92.

[9] Global Action Plan for the Prevention and Control of Noncommunicable Diseases 2013–2020, WHA66.10, 27 May 2013, http://apps.who.int/gb/ebwha/pdf_files/WHA66/A66_R10-en.pdf.

[10] Global Code of Practice on the International Recruitment of Health Personnel, WHA63.16, 21 May 2010, http://apps.who.int/gb/ebwha/pdf_files/WHA63/A63_R16-en.pdf.

[11] Review of the Constitution and Regional Arrangements of the World Health Organization, EB101/7, 14 November 1997, http://apps.who.int/gb/archive/pdf_files/EB101/pdfangl/eb1017.pdf.

[12] World Health Organization, *Primary Health Care: Report of the International Conference on Primary Health Care, Alma-Ata, USSR, 6–12 September 1978*, Geneva, 1978, http://whqlibdoc.who.int/publications/9241800011.pdf.

[13] The Ottawa Charter for Health Promotion, http://www.who.int/healthpromotion/conferences/previous/ottawa/en/.

[14] The 8th Global Conference on Health Promotion, Helsinki, Finland, 10–14 June 2013. The Helsinki statement on Health in All Policies, http://www.who.int/healthpromotion/conferences/8gchp/statement_2013/en.

[15] Reducing Health Inequities through Action on the Social Determinants of Health, WHA62.14, 22 May 2009, http://apps.who.int/gb/ebwha/pdf_files/A62/A62_R14-en.pdf.

[16] Climate Change and Health, WHA61.19, 24 May 2008, http://www.who.int/globalchange/A61_R19_en.pdf.

than a decade.[17] The relationship between trade and health has been placed on the WHO's agenda but has not been actively pursued, although the potential impact of the many planned and actual trade and investment agreements on public health is increasingly a cause for concern.[18] Yet again, the resources that the WHO has been able to devote to these areas has been minimal. The current debate on the shape of the post-2015 development agenda and on the proper place of health in the sustainable development agenda is also, by implication, a debate about the appropriate role for the WHO in promoting better health in current world circumstances, and the overall balance to be struck between improving health services and addressing the economic, social and environmental determinants of health.

How the WHO should address these inter-sectoral issues that affect health has never been properly resolved. The WHO's historical focus has been on tackling – or sometimes eliminating – specific diseases, but today's view of health is more holistic. On the one hand, there is a focus on ways in which health systems, as opposed to specific disease programmes, should be developed and strengthened. On the other hand, there is recognition of how health status has been profoundly affected by social, economic and environmental factors, and also by political processes outside the health sector. These arise particularly as a result of the massive increase in social and economic inequalities linked to globalization and economic transformation in emerging economies. A recent commission set out the need to address the political determinants of health that lie outside the health sector. Interestingly, however, in proposing new mechanisms for coordination, it passed over the WHO as a central player because, in its words:

> It has so far not been able to open up space and arenas for policy dialogue inclusive of other relevant intergovernmental organisations, governments, and non-state actors […] This situation has limited the effectiveness of WHO, making it unable to coordinate a coherent approach that unites political and public will and private sector readiness to act on necessary policies and regulations.[19]

New global health institutions

The health gains of the recent past are mainly the result of efforts by countries, but are also partially attributable to the rapid increase in development assistance for health,

which has increased more than fivefold in real terms since 1990.[20] Progress in fighting the big three diseases – AIDS, tuberculosis and malaria – has particularly benefited from expanded flows of international assistance. Accompanying this has been the rise of new institutions and new funding mechanisms that, in the eyes of many, have challenged the WHO's role as a directing and coordinating authority.

These new governance structures have highlighted the difficulties that the WHO has in incorporating non-governmental stakeholders constructively into its consultative and deliberative activities.

The substantial challenge began with the entry of the World Bank into health-sector lending on a large scale in the 1980s, and subsequently with the creation of UNAIDS in 1994/95 and the International AIDS Vaccine Initiative (IAVI) in 1996, the latter being the first public–private partnership devoted to product development. Since 2000, however, there has been a burgeoning of new institutions developed to tackle specific disease problems. These include the GAVI Alliance (formerly the Global Alliance for Vaccines and Immunisation), the Global Fund to Fight AIDS, Tuberculosis and Malaria (the Global Fund) and UNITAID, the international drug purchase facility. A host of new public–private partnerships for product development has arisen, such as the Medicines for Malaria Venture (MMV) or Drugs for Neglected Diseases initiative (DNDi), along with new private-sector actors such as the Bill & Melinda Gates Foundation. In addition, there have been bilateral initiatives of global significance, such as the US President's Emergency Plan for AIDS Relief (PEPFAR).

A characteristic of these new global institutions is new forms of governance, in particular the inclusion of representatives of civil society, the private sector and foundations in the governance mechanisms. This contrasts with the largely intergovernmental nature of UN organizations, notably the WHO, in which member states jealously guard the prerogative of governments in decision-making. These new governance structures have highlighted the difficulties that the WHO has in incorporating non-governmental stakeholders constructively into its consultative and deliberative activities.

[17] 'WHO Director-General addresses meeting on the financing and coordination of R&D', 26 November 2012, http://www.who.int/dg/speeches/2012/cewg_20121126/en/index.html.

[18] International Trade and Health, WHA59.26, 27 May 2006, https://apps.who.int/gb/ebwha/pdf_files/WHA59/A59_R26-en.pdf.

[19] 'The Political Origins of Health Inequity: Prospects for Change', The Lancet–University of Oslo Commission on Global Governance for Health, *The Lancet*, Vol. 383, 15 February 2014, http://download.thelancet.com/pdfs/journals/lancet/PIIS0140673613624071.pdf.

[20] *Financing Global Health 2013: Transition in an Age of Austerity*, Institute of Health Metrics and Evaluation. April 2014, http://www.healthmetricsandevaluation.org/sites/default/files/policy_report/2014/IHME_FGH2013_Overview.pdf.

Some are also concerned that health-related subjects are dealt with in New York rather than in Geneva. In recent times, for instance, the UN General Assembly has adopted resolutions on non-communicable diseases[21] and on universal health coverage.[22] On the other hand, both resolutions recognize the leading role of the WHO in the UN system in dealing with these issues.

The WHO's reform programme

Meanwhile, the WHO's secure funding from governments has stagnated, and it has become overwhelmingly reliant on voluntary contributions from governments and other funders – usually earmarked for particular activities favoured by the donor. The Bill & Melinda Gates Foundation has in the space of one decade become the single biggest voluntary contributor to the WHO. Indeed by 2013 the foundation was the WHO's largest funder, providing $301 million, which exceeded the United States' combined voluntary and assessed contributions of $290 million.[23]

This reliance on uncertain and inflexible sources of funding was the principal reason why in January 2010 WHO Director-General Margaret Chan initiated what has become a determined effort to reform how the organization functions. As a result, discussions in the WHO's governance bodies over the last four years have been dominated by this issue.

In introducing the informal consultation on the future of financing for the WHO, Chan identified two key issues:

- how better to align the priorities agreed by the WHO's governing bodies with the monies available to finance them; and

- how to ensure greater predictability and stability of financing to promote more realistic planning and effective management.

The report of that meeting noted that while the WHO's financing was the starting point for the consultation, it prompted a series of more fundamental questions about what should constitute the WHO's core business. How, for instance, should the mandate to 'act as the directing and co-ordinating authority on international health work' be understood in the radically changed landscape in which the WHO now operated, more than 60 years after its constitution was drafted?

Questions that emerged in the consultation included:

- To what extent, and how, should the WHO address the broader social and economic determinants of health?

- What constitutes good partnership behaviour at the global and country level – and what are the implications for the WHO?

- What constitutes effective country support in countries at very different levels of development and capacity – and how can the WHO match the support it provides more closely and flexibly to country needs?

- How can the WHO be more consistent and effective in the field of technical collaboration?[24]

The WHO's reform programme has now become institutionalized around the themes of programmes and priority-setting, governance and managerial reform. This report also addresses these themes. There are many questions about how the WHO should locate itself in relation to this new and crowded institutional environment for global health. How should it interpret or reinterpret its constitutional role? As an organization principally composed of medical and health professionals, how can it effectively address the social, economic, environmental and political determinants of health? As an intergovernmental organization, how can it effectively engage with these new actors, including NGOs, charitable foundations and the private sector? As an organization with half its staff in country offices, and a quarter in regional offices, what does it need to do at regional and country level that cannot, or should not, be done by others?

Difficult issues avoided

The working group considered that the current reform programme as it has unfolded has not dealt in any great depth with a number of fundamental issues because, as noted above, although of great importance they are politically difficult to deal with. The WHO, like any other institution, has grown up in a way that creates groups which are likely to feel threatened by change. The reforms attempted under the leadership of former Director-General Gro Harlem Brundtland provide a good illustration of such a reaction.[25]

[21] Political Declaration of the High-level Meeting of the General Assembly on the Prevention and Control of Non-communicable Diseases. A/RES/66/2, 24 January 2012, http://www.who.int/nmh/events/un_ncd_summit2011/political_declaration_en.pdf?ua=1.

[22] Global Health and Foreign Policy, A/67/L.36, 6 December 2012, http://www.un.org/ga/search/viewm_doc.asp?symbol=A/67/L.36.

[23] Annex to the Financial Report and Audited Financial Statements for the year ended 31 December 2013, Voluntary contributions by fund and by contributor, 17 April 2014. Assessed contribution payable summary for 2012–2013, http://www.who.int/about/resources_planning/2012_2013_AC_summary.pdf?ua=1.

[24] *The Future of Financing for WHO: Report of an Informal Consultation Convened by the Director-General*, Geneva, Switzerland, 12–13 January 2010, http://www.who.int/about/resources_planning/AnnexA67-43-en.pdf?ua=1f.

[25] Clift, C., 'The Role of the World Health Organization in the International System', Working Group Paper, Chatham House, February 2013, http://www.chathamhouse.org/publications/papers/view/189351.

In the extensive documentation about the WHO reform process made available by the Secretariat since 2010,[26] and in all the discussions within the WHO's governing bodies, the Executive Board (EB) and the World Health Assembly (WHA), since then, there are key issues that are not discussed, or not discussed with any rigour. Outside commentators, including some who previously worked for the WHO, provide a completely different perspective on what is wrong with the organization. For example, a former assistant director-general viewed the problem as follows:

> The WHO – for 62 years the world's go-to agency on all public health matters – is today outmoded, underfunded, and overly politicized. In a world of rapid technological change, travel, and trade, the WHO moves with a bureaucracy's speed. Its advice to health officials is too often muddied by the need for consensus. Regional leadership posts are pursued as political prizes. Underfunded and over strapped, the organization has come under attack for being too easily swayed by big pharma. In a world where foundations, NGOs, and the private sector are transforming global health, the WHO has simply not adapted. This isn't just about the WHO losing its edge. Taken together, these myriad dysfunctions are rendering the WHO closer and closer to irrelevancy in the world of global health.[27]

This is no doubt overstated for effect and lacks coherence as a critique, but it nevertheless highlights some of the most common criticisms that are raised when the woes of the WHO are discussed by those who work for it, or interact frequently with it: that it is

- Over-politicized to the detriment of its technical functions;
- Too bureaucratic;
- Timid;
- Overstretched/underfunded;
- Conflicted; and
- Failing to adapt to change.

Overall, there is the perception that the WHO, in this changed world, and as a result of the above deficiencies, has failed to identify its proper role in the governance of global health. It does not seem appropriate today that the WHO should have a directing – as opposed to a coordinating – role, if it ever did; but the need for coordination with the multiplicity of new actors and stakeholders in global health is possibly much greater than in the past. Yet the WHO and its member states have hitherto failed to get to grips with what that role really should be.

Furthermore, any conversation about the WHO rapidly turns to its unique structure – with six regional offices, the members of which, through a regional committee composed of member states, elect their own regional director (RD) – and how this configuration affects the effectiveness, efficiency and coherence of the WHO as an organization.

As early as 1993 the independent Joint Inspection Unit (JIU) of the UN noted that 'while the three-layer organizational structure appears excellent as described in the Constitution and official documents, its actual functioning is beset by serious and complex problems of a constitutional, political, managerial and programmatic nature'.[28] It identified the way in which RDs were elected by their regional committees as the central problem. But the JIU's proposals, seeking to depoliticize the regional committees by reasserting the authority of the EB and the director-general in the appointment of RDs, were not taken up by the EB.

A further review by the JIU, commissioned in 2012 as part of the current reform programme, largely endorsed the findings of the 1993 report, but accepted the current director-general's view that the same objective could be achieved by better teamwork and creating a culture of 'One WHO' without changing role of the director-general in the selection process for RDs.[29] Nevertheless, it concluded that the regional committees were largely ineffective in providing oversight of the work of regional offices, and that the 'Executive Board should complete, in the context of the current WHO reform process, a comprehensive review of the governance process at regional level and put forward concrete proposals to improve the functioning of Regional Committees and subcommittees'. In response, the EB simply asked the director-general to take account of the recommendations of the JIU report in implementing the reform programme – in all probability to bury it in the myriad of ongoing issues in WHO reform.[30]

As regards the WHO's 150 country offices, a very similar pattern of resistance to change emerges. In 1997, following a donor-financed study of country offices,[31] the WHO

---

[26] WHO Reform Process: Documents, http://www.who.int/about/who_reform/documents.

[27] Chow, J., 'Is the WHO Becoming Irrelevant?', *Foreign Policy*, 8 December 2010, http://www.foreignpolicy.com/articles/2010/12/08/is_the_who_becoming_irrelevant.

[28] Joint Inspection Unit, 'Decentralization of Organizations within the United Nations System. Part III: The World Health Organization', Geneva, 1993, https://www.unjiu.org/en/reports-notes/JIU%20Products/JIU_REP_1993_2_ENGLISH.pdf.

[29] Review of Management, Administration and Decentralization in the World Health Organization', Joint Inspection Unit, Geneva, 2012, E132/5 Add.6, 4 January 2013, http://apps.who.int/gb/ebwha/pdf_files/EB132/B132_5Add6-en.pdf.

[30] Decisions and List of Resolutions, EB132/DIV./3, 26 February 2013, http://apps.who.int/gb/ebwha/pdf_files/EB132/B132_DIV3-en.pdf.

[31] Lucas, A. et al., 'Cooperation for Health Development: The World Health Organization's Support to Programmes at Country Level', September 1997, http://whqlibdoc.who.int/publications/0N02657577_V1_(ch1-ch2).pdf.http://whqlibdoc.who.int/publications/0N02657577_V1_(ch1-ch2).pdf; 'Cooperation for Health Development: WHO's Support to Programmes at Country Level. Summary', September 1997, http://www.norad.no/en/tools-and-publications/publications/publication?key=109668.

Secretariat put to the EB quite radical proposals for country office reform.[32] The premise of this report was that the WHO, faced by severely constrained finances, needed to focus its country-level support on fulfilling the needs of least developed countries. It recommended that more successful developing countries should be encouraged to meet the costs, partially or wholly, of their WHO country office. In addition, as health and economic status improved, some countries should no longer require a country office. Other mechanisms could be considered to maintain a WHO presence in these countries, such as shared offices, liaison offices or special representatives to deal with a set of countries or activities. Moreover, the cost of the country office should not be treated as part of the country allocation for technical support and assistance – thus avoiding penalizing countries that agreed to a reduced WHO presence. Where countries resisted a request for reduced WHO presence, they should be obliged to meet the costs of that presence. By grouping countries according to their health and economic status, the report identified a large number of more advanced developing countries where alternative or less costly arrangements for WHO representation should be considered.

The 2013 evaluation notes that the WHO 'has not addressed with enough vigour the question of its role in global health governance'.

But little or no substantive action followed. In 2001 a JIU report on WHO management criticized the lack of progress, and recommended that the director-general 'should finalize as a matter of priority the common set of objective criteria called for by the EB to determine the nature and extent of WHO country representation'.[33] Again, nothing happened. The 2012 JIU follow-up report (referred to above) noted – apparently with frustration – that no action had been taken on the recommendation of its 2001 report, which it still believed to be necessary.[34] The EB reaction to the 2012 JIU report recommendations was as reported above – i.e. to ask the director-general to take account of JIU recommendations in implementing the reform programme. Further comments in the same vein in the 2013 evaluation of the reform programme commissioned by the WHO from PwC (henceforth '2013 evaluation') have to date produced no reaction from member states or the Secretariat.[35]

Apart from the regional and country structure, which absorbs more than 60 per cent of the WHO's resources, an issue that has been addressed to some extent in the internal reform programme, but that has proved intractable, is that of the WHO's role in global health governance – both in respect of its partner institutions and stakeholders in the health sector ('governance of health') and in relationships with actors outside the health sector whose policies and decisions have an impact on health ('governance for health'). So this is an issue that has not been entirely avoided, but in which member states have failed to grasp the nettle of what role they want the WHO to play in both these aspects of global health governance. The 2013 evaluation notes that the WHO 'has not addressed with enough vigour the question of its role in global health governance'.[36]

The political economy of reform

The above illustrates very well the way in which difficult decisions relating to the structure of the WHO are not addressed by member states, simply because they do not consider it in their interest to do so. As one member pointed out in the context of a discussion on changing the status of regional offices:

> the people sitting around the regional committees often have a personal stake in the regional office being there, because it's a retirement job for them, or it's a promotion for them, or it's a job when they get kicked out of government. And you're asking those people to vote themselves out of a job.

And another, with particular reference to the reform of country offices:

> these are staff positions that are being centrally paid by Geneva so of course every country is going to guard their country office vigorously. And beyond that the WR [WHO Representative] office has many [...] national professional officers there, and many senior people in the ministry of health are waiting to get the WR office jobs or even regional office jobs. And these are the people who will vote to abolish WR offices, regional offices. Will that happen while they are waiting in line to get into that? Because once you are in WHO your kids can go to world class universities with 70–75% paid by WHO. You have all the benefits. You are like the rat falling into a rice pot.

These quotations illustrate how the financing mechanisms of the WHO predispose developing-country member states to favour the status quo. They pay a relatively small assessed contribution to the WHO, in return for which they have access to the services and job opportunities offered by the

[32] *WHO Reform. WHO Country Offices. Report by the Director-General*, EB101/5, 4 December 1997, http://apps.who.int/gb/archive/pdf_files/EB101/pdfangl/ang5.pdf.
[33] Review of Management and Administration in the World Health Organization. Joint Inspection Unit. Geneva, 2001. https://www.unjiu.org/en/reports-notes/archive/JIU_REP_2001_5_English.pdf.
[34] Review of Management, Administration and Decentralization in the World Health Organization. Joint Inspection Unit, Geneva, 2012. E132/5 Add.6. 4 January 2013. http://apps.who.int/gb/ebwha/pdf_files/EB132/B132_5Add6-en.pdf.
[35] Second Stage Evaluation on WHO Reform. EB134/39. 3 January 2014. http://apps.who.int/gb/ebwha/pdf_files/EB134/B134_39-en.pdf.
[36] Ibid.

regional and country offices. Thus high-income countries, as classified by the World Bank, contributed in 2012/13 about 88 per cent of the total assessed contributions to the WHO.[37] All other countries therefore contributed about 12 per cent, or about $115 million, compared with the WHO's expenditure of $2.7 billion on regional and country offices in the same biennium. To take an extreme example, Nigeria's assessed contribution in 2012/2013 was $725,000, in return for which it benefits from the WHO's largest country office of nearly 350 people at a biennial cost of about $72 million, as well as the services offered by the African regional office, the WHO's largest.[38]

The working group noted that the politicization affected the organization in myriad harmful ways. This was particularly the case in relation to elections and appointments at headquarters, the regions and countries, where politics and patronage may mean appointments are made on grounds other than merit. Commenting under the Chatham House Rule some members described the use of payments and other inducements to EB and regional committee members at election times. For example, concerns about this were widely aired when Hiroshi Nakajima was reappointed director-general in 1993.[39] It was also concern about the RD election process that led the Western Pacific Regional Office (WPRO) in 2012 to introduce a code of conduct for nomination of an RD, the first example of such a code in any UN organization.[40]

However, politicization is not just about electioneering: it throws a long shadow over the way in which the organization as a whole operates. The notorious slowness of decision-making in the WHO is in large part a result of its complex structure, which necessitates the negotiation of decisions between departments and between the different levels of the organization, any of which may do things differently for a variety of reasons other than technical considerations. The WHO is unique in that bureaucratic politics – common in any large organization, particularly international ones – is overlaid with politics deriving from the fact that regional leadership owes its principal allegiance to ministries of health in the region which elect it, rather than to the director-general in Geneva.

Although many in the working group personally favoured reform of the regional structure in principle, one view in the group was that reform that touched on the regional and country office structure, even if desirable, was simply politically unrealistic because of the entrenched nature of the status quo. This is essentially the stance adopted in the current internal WHO reform process: the current regional and country set-up is more or less taken as a given, although lip service is paid to the need to make improvements. Others in the group felt, for a combination of reasons, that because change would inevitably be contentious and potentially disruptive in the short term, the benefits of reform needed to be assessed pragmatically against the costs of both action and inaction. That a course of action was in principle desirable did not mean that it was necessarily wise to pursue it.

It was felt that the group must draw appropriate conclusions from the history of failed reform attempts in the WHO; otherwise, nothing much would happen yet again. While the internal dynamics of the governance institutions in the WHO militated against changes to the status quo, there are nevertheless significant constituencies both within the WHO and among its stakeholders who support the need for change. However, the members of these constituencies, arguably more numerous than supporters of the status quo, were not politically empowered. Ultimately, real change could only be brought about in the WHO if its principal funders desired it sufficiently to put up with the aggravation that bringing about change would necessarily entail.

There is quite a lot of evidence – not least the absence of real change – that the main funders of the WHO have long been prepared to settle for a second-best situation, rather than dirtying their hands with the messy business of reform. In the words of our background paper:

> Although the functioning of WHO had been reviewed in various ways from its very early days, serious consideration of the need for reform began in the late 1980s and early 1990s, stimulated in part by more general concerns about the whole UN system. These had become evident long before in 1964 when the Geneva Group of 11 major contributors to the UN was formed to restrain the growth of agency budgets.[41] By 1984 they had largely achieved the aim of restricting the growth of agency budgets to zero in real terms, including for WHO. The use of this blunt instrument was a reflection of the difficulty in achieving changes in performance and accountability of the UN system, so budget restriction was the second-best policy in their eyes. Paradoxically this simply shifted donor interest to ways in which they could achieve their objectives for WHO through voluntary contributions usually earmarked for the pursuit of particular programmes they promoted or favoured.[42]

There has always been a tension between the WHO's role as a standard-setter (its normative function) and as a provider of technical assistance and support to developing countries.

[37] Assessed Contribution Payable Summary for 2012–2013, http://www.who.int/about/resources_planning/2012_2013_AC_summary.pdf?ua=1.

[38] 'WHO Reform. Programmes and Priority Setting: Summary Information on the Distribution of Financial and Human Resources to Each Level and Cluster', EB130/5 Add.2, 13 January 2012, http://apps.who.int/gb/ebwha/pdf_files/EB130/B130_5Add2-en.pdf.

[39] 'Payments linked to election for WHO leader', *New York Times,* 20 February 1993. http://www.nytimes.com/1993/02/20/world/payments-linked-to-election-for-who-leader.html; 'West decries re-election of WHO chief', *New York Times, 22* January 1993, http://www.nytimes.com/1993/01/22/news/22iht-who__0.html.

[40] Nomination of the Regional Director: Code of Conduct, Resolution WPR/RC63.R7, 27 September 2012, http://www.wpro.who.int/about/regional_committee/63/resolutions/WPR_RC63_R7_RD_Nomination_code_of_conduct_complete_with_annex.pdf.

[41] Overseas Development Institute, 'The UN and the Future of Multilateralism', Briefing Paper, London, October 1987, http://www.odi.org.uk/resources/docs/6728.pdf.

[42] Clift, 'The Role of the World Health Organization in the International System'.

Historically, developed countries represented in the WHO's governance structures by their health or foreign affairs ministries have tended to see most value in its normative functions. By contrast, developing countries in the WHO have emphasized its technical assistance and support role. In the 1970s the WHA passed a resolution demanding that 60 per cent of the regular budget be allocated for this purpose.[43] Thus, for a variety of reasons based on strategic and personal interest considerations, developing countries tend to support the status quo within the WHO. And to some extent they are supported by the voluntary contributors to the WHO (both member-state development agencies and others) who, while often questioning the WHO's overall efficiency, nevertheless value its extensive country network as a vehicle for delivering projects.

Conclusion

The working group contested the mythology of a 'golden age' in which the WHO actually performed the function of being the directing and coordinating body in international health. According to this mythology, the history of the WHO has been one of a downward slide in which it has gradually lost its erstwhile authority, which has passed to the multitude of other global health agencies outlined above. In this view, the very existence of organizations such as GAVI or the Global Fund is a reminder of the WHO's failure, and of the extent to which the international community (particularly the donor community) prefers to bypass a WHO that is perceived as clodhopping and ineffective.

Nevertheless, the group was very clear that the WHO had never been intended as a body that should undertake each and every function that might contribute to global health. It was not meant to be a funding agency, nor indeed a research organization. Praise rather than blame should attach to it for promoting and fostering new institutions to fund health service provision or to undertake research (for instance MMV).

Moreover, the new and more complex institutional structure in global health, which accompanied the increase in funding, was also to be welcomed. While there were drawbacks to this proliferation of funding bodies, notably the increased transactions costs for countries responding to the uncoordinated demands of multiple donors, the new infrastructure had also offered more choice for countries seeking funding or technical assistance and innovation in governance structures as well as in funding methods. An element of competition to traditional providers such as the World Bank and the WHO was, on balance, considered a good thing.[44]

It was open to serious question whether the WHO should in practice seek to direct work in international health, as provided for in its constitution. The idea that it was a directing authority led too frequently to a mindset within the WHO that others should conform to its way of doing things, and in several cases this has undermined its ability to forge effective partnerships with others.

On the other hand, the very same proliferation of global health institutions surely provided the opportunity for the WHO to make more of its coordinating function as specified in the constitution: providing leadership, offering guidance and promoting coherence between the many different actors. Similarly, the WHO surely had a role to play in influencing other actors within and outside the health sector – both governmental and non-governmental – to behave in ways that sought to reconcile the political, economic and commercial objectives of these actors with public health goals.

In the light of all this, the group considered that the current process of reform should be used as an opportunity for the WHO and its member states to think how it should reposition itself in current circumstances as a leader in global health. This needs to be based on a proper analysis of what the WHO's role should be in relation to the health challenges now confronting the world.

The rest of this report seeks to define what that role should be, and what this means for the WHO's governance, financing and management.

[43] Programme Budget Policy, WHA29.48, 17 May 1976, http://hist.library.paho.org/english/GOV/CD/26340.pdf.
[44] Blanchet, N. et al., 'Global Collective Action in Health: The WDR+20 Landscape of Core and Supportive Functions', Working Paper for The Lancet Commission on Investing in Health, 5 July 2013, http://globalhealth2035.org/sites/default/files/working-papers/global-collective-action-in-health.pdf; Hoffman, S. and Røttingen, J.-A., 'Global Health Governance after 2015', The Lancet, Vol. 382 (2013), 9897: 1018, http://www.thelancet.com/journals/lancet/article/PIIS0140-6736(13)61966-2/fulltext.

2. What Should the WHO Do?

Introduction

The working group's consideration of the WHO's role was influenced by a framework proposed in 1998 as a means of analysing the functions that an international health body should perform.[45] In this framework, there are two groups of functions that may be appropriate for international collective action.

Core functions are those relating to necessary areas of collective action that individual nation-states could not undertake alone. These have the nature of what we now call global public goods that would otherwise be undersupplied. They include, for instance, guidelines and protocols setting out best clinical practice; setting norms and standards; maintaining the International Classification of Diseases; collective agreements such as the International Health Regulations (IHR) or the FCTC; coordinating international action to combat pandemics or control diseases, and providing a global forum to harness global expertise. Core functions are required equally by rich and poor nations because they are correcting a form of 'market failure'. Every nation can experience better health and better health security through the exercise of collective action in these areas.

> **Core functions are required equally by rich and poor nations because they are correcting a form of 'market failure'. Every nation can experience better health and better health security through the exercise of collective action.**

By contrast, *supportive functions* are those that are carried out internationally for a number of reasons (e.g. humanitarian or altruistic), but are essentially to support governments to undertake functions that should be undertaken nationally but which, for one reason or another, governments are unable to carry out adequately themselves. Development aid for health is the principal example of a supportive action. The authors characterized these functions as compensating for 'government failure'. The need for international support varies inversely with economic circumstances.

The authors of the 1998 framework considered that the WHO's primary functions lay in the core domain, whereas those of the World Bank or UNICEF, for example, lay in the supportive domain. Recent elaborations of this framework, taking account of the proliferation of new funders and new institutions in global health since 1998, note that the great majority of the increase in funding for health has been to supportive functions (through organizations such as the World Bank, GAVI and PEPFAR); and this applies also to the WHO, where voluntary contributions have been the main source of budgetary growth. The expectation in 1998 had been that supportive funding would decrease relative to 'core' funding for global public goods. This carries the implication that the functions of the WHO as a provider of global public goods and as a steward of the overall global health system have been neglected and its energies have been dissipated in the supply of supportive services that may be better suited to supply by other bodies.[46]

WHO functions

The constitution

The working group spent some time considering what might be considered the WHO's core functions in terms of the 22 listed in the constitution – i.e. the tasks that only the WHO rather than another agency could undertake. A list of nine functions (italicized in Box 1) was tentatively identified, but it was felt that the exercise was not very helpful. By definition, it was legitimate for the WHO to be involved in any activity covered by the constitution, which, given the last, catch-all function, was not constrained in any way.

This was one of the WHO's key problems: the boundaries of the activities that it could legitimately pursue were undefined. An internal report on resource mobilization noted:

> WHO lacks a clear grasp of its comparative advantage, including at country level, at times taking on what others might do better. Its core mandate and functions are so broadly formulated that the boundaries of operation become invisible. It is up to individual offices and programmes to decide what to take on [...] WHO is to a large extent driven by funding opportunities and is spread too thinly. It has too many priorities, everything being a priority. It is unable to terminate projects and therefore tends to become unfocused, reinventing and repackaging rather than concluding, learning and inventing.[47]

---

[45] Jamison, D. et al., 'International Collective Action in Health: Objectives, Functions, and Rationale', *The Lancet*, 351 (1998): 514–17, http://www.bvsde.paho.org/texcom/cd050852/jamison.pdf.

[46] Frenk, J. and Moon, S., 'Governance Challenges in Global Health', *New England Journal of Medicine* (2013), 368: 936–42, http://www.nejm.org/doi/full/10.1056/NEJMra1109339.

[47] 'Task Force on Resource Mobilization and Management Strategies. Situation and Diagnosis', World Health Organization, 2013, http://www.who.int/about/who_reform/TFRMMS-report-annex-2013.pdf?ua=1.

Box 1: Article 2 of the WHO constitution: functions of the WHO

In order to achieve its objective, the functions of the Organization shall be:

a. *to act as the directing and co-ordinating authority on international health work;*

b. *to establish and maintain effective collaboration with the United Nations, specialized agencies, governmental health administrations, professional groups and such other organizations as may be deemed appropriate;*[a]

c. to assist Governments, upon request, in strengthening health services;

d. *to furnish appropriate technical assistance and, in emergencies, necessary aid upon the request or acceptance of Governments;*

e. to provide or assist in providing, upon the request of the United Nations, health services and facilities to special groups, such as the peoples of trust territories;

f. *to establish and maintain such administrative and technical services as may be required, including epidemiological and statistical services;*

g. to stimulate and advance work to eradicate epidemic, endemic and other diseases;

h. to promote, in co-operation with other specialized agencies where necessary, the prevention of accidental injuries;

i. to promote, in co-operation with other specialized agencies where necessary, the improvement of nutrition, housing, sanitation, recreation, economic or working conditions and other aspects of environmental hygiene;

j. to promote co-operation among scientific and professional groups which contribute to the advancement of health;

k. *to propose conventions, agreements and regulations, and make recommendations with respect to international health matters*

and to perform such duties as may be assigned thereby to the Organization and are consistent with its objective;

l. to promote maternal and child health and welfare and to foster the ability to live harmoniously in a changing total environment;

m. to foster activities in the field of mental health, especially those affecting the harmony of human relations;

n. to promote and conduct research in the field of health;

o. to promote improved standards of teaching and training in the health, medical and related professions;

p. to study and report on, in co-operation with other specialized agencies where necessary, administrative and social techniques affecting public health and medical care from preventive and curative points of view, including hospital services and social security;

q. to provide information, counsel and assistance in the field of health;

r. to assist in developing an informed public opinion among all peoples on matters of health;

s. *to establish and revise as necessary international nomenclatures of diseases, of causes of death and of public health practices;*

t. *to standardize diagnostic procedures as necessary;*

u. *to develop, establish and promote international standards with respect to food, biological, pharmaceutical and similar products;*

v. *generally to take all necessary action to attain the objective of the Organization.*

---

[a] The working group considered this might now refer explicitly to 'civil society, foundations and the private sector'.

Source: The WHO Constitution, http://www.who.int/governance/eb/who_constitution_en.pdf.
Note: Italicized paragraphs are those that the group considered wholly or partially core.

New issues

The working group also noted that there were a number of 'new' issues that had become prominent since 1948. Some were partly envisaged in the list of WHO functions or in the preamble to the constitution, but have achieved more prominence in subsequent health debates than envisaged by many at the time. Although the importance of other economic and social sectors to health status is partly reflected in the constitution, the issue of how the WHO – as an agency staffed principally by health professionals – should address the health implications of actions in other sectors is a perennial source of unresolved debate. This applies, for instance, in relation to the stream of work arising from the report of the 2008 Commission on the Social Determinants of Health[48] or (a subject not anticipated in 1948) climate change.[49]

---

[48] Reducing Health Inequities through Action on the Social Determinants of Health. Resolution WHA 62.14, 22 May 2009, http://apps.who.int/gb/ebwha/pdf_files/WHA62-REC1/WHA62_REC1-en-P2.pdf.
[49] Climate Change and Health, Resolution WHA61.19, 24 May 2008, http://apps.who.int/gb/ebwha/pdf_files/A61/A61_R19-en.pdf?ua=1.

Another 'new' subject not contemplated explicitly in the constitution is the issue of the coherence between trade and health policies, including the impact of intellectual property rights on innovation and access to health care. The WHO was asked in 2006 to support member states to frame coherent policies and build capacity to understand the implications of trade agreements for health and to develop appropriate policies and legislation accordingly; and to support policy coherence between the trade and health sectors, including generating and sharing evidence on the relationship between trade and health.[50] In reality, the WHO has been unable to do a significant amount of work in this area since 2006, despite the growing controversy about the impact of proposed and existing trade agreements on health. The parallel stream of work on intellectual property, initiated in the 1990s, has been long-lived and unresolved, principally because member states are divided about the extent to which intellectual property rights are a proper subject for the WHO in terms of its health mandate. Furthermore, underlying that argument is a division between member states who regard the existing intellectual property regime as integral to their economic and political interests and those who see it, to a greater or lesser extent, as a potential obstacle to economic development and a threat to public health through limiting access to affordable medicines.

Working group analysis

The context for considering what role the WHO should play is that it is insufficiently financed to execute many of the functions that it is mandated to undertake. This is why the WHO embarked on a process of internal reform, and is why choices need to be made about what is it essential that the WHO does and what others can do equally well. Such choices need to be made in the context of the resources likely to be available to the WHO, and the predictability and sustainability of these resources. The working group did not agree that the WHO was underfinanced: rather that there was scope for doing less, but better and more efficiently. It was also aware that because of the predominance of earmarked voluntary contributions in the WHO's budget, decisions on cutting out particular functions may not automatically – or even at all – result in additional resources for retained functions because the resources are tied to particular activities. For example, in the current programme budget $700 million is allocated to the Global Polio Eradication Initiative which finances over 1,000 of the

WHO's 7,000 staff and over 6,000 further personnel on non-staff contracts. The organization is currently considering the implications of the planned completion of the initiative in 2018.[51]

As the WHO itself says:

> WHO continues to play a critical role as the world's leading technical authority on health. At the same time, the Organization has found itself overcommitted, overextended and in need of reform. Priority setting, in particular, has been neither sufficiently selective nor strategically focused. Moreover, most analysts now suggest that the financial crisis will have long term consequences, and not only in the OECD countries that provide a large proportion of WHO's voluntary funding. It is therefore evident that WHO needs to respond strategically to a new, longer term constrained financial reality rather than reacting managerially to a short term crisis. Sustainable and predictable financing that is aligned to a carefully defined set of priorities, and agreed by Member States, is therefore central to the vision of a reformed WHO.[52]

After due deliberation, the working group considered that the core functions that the WHO has defined in its current General Programme of Work (GPW) are a reasonable basis for proceeding. They are:

- Providing leadership on matters critical to health and engaging in partnerships where joint action is needed;

- Shaping the research agenda and stimulating the generation, translation and dissemination of valuable knowledge;

- Setting norms and standards, and promoting and monitoring their implementation;

- Articulating ethical and evidence-based policy options;

- Providing technical support, catalysing change, and building sustainable institutional capacity;

- Monitoring the health situation and assessing health trends.[53]

One question is whether these functions adequately reflect the WHO's role in public health emergencies such as pandemics. The working group thought there should be a general function related to the WHO's role in promoting and maintaining global health security. For instance, this would cover the 'preparedness, surveillance and response' category in the programme budget, which includes the WHO's response to disease outbreaks, acute public health emergencies and the effective management of health-related aspects of humanitarian disasters in order to

---

[50] International Trade and Health. Resolution WHA 59.26 27 May 2006, http://apps.who.int/gb/ebwha/pdf_files/WHA59-REC1/e/Resolutions-en.pdf.
[51] Human Resources: Annual Report, A67/47, 17 April 2014, http://apps.who.int/gb/ebwha/pdf_files/WHA67/A67_47-en.pdf.
[52] Draft twelfth general programme of work. A66/6, 19 April 2013, http://apps.who.int/gb/ebwha/pdf_files/WHA66/A66_6-en.pdf.
[53] Ibid.

contribute to health security. This also includes the WHO's work on implementing the IHR, pandemic and emergency preparedness, and polio eradication. So a seventh function might be:

- Promoting and maintaining global health security.

Similarly, as referred to above, the WHO's technical assistance role needs to be restricted to those things that can best be done by the WHO, rather than other agencies. In this sense, its technical assistance functions should be related to the WHO's role as a provider of global public goods. This is discussed further below and in Chapter 4.

Except inasmuch as leadership and partnerships are all-encompassing, the functions also do not refer explicitly to the WHO's leadership role in relation to the global governance of health (in relation to its coordinating function in respect of other health sector actors), or to its role in relation to global governance for health (as regards the impact of decisions and actions in other sectors that affect health). The WHO elaborates the following leadership priorities as 'intended emphases […] highlighting where the WHO aims to enhance visibility and to shape the global conversation, extending its role in global health governance':

- **Advancing universal health coverage:** enabling countries to sustain or expand access to essential health services and financial protection and promoting universal health coverage as a unifying concept in global health.

- **Health-related Millennium Development Goals:** addressing unfinished and future challenges: accelerating the achievement of the current health-related goals up to and beyond 2015. This priority includes completing the eradication of polio and selected neglected tropical diseases.

- **Addressing the challenge of non-communicable diseases** and mental health, violence and injuries and disabilities.

- Implementing the provisions of the **International Health Regulations:** ensuring that all countries can meet the capacity requirements specified in the International Health Regulations (2005).

- Increasing access to essential, high-quality and affordable **medical products** (medicines, vaccines, diagnostics and other health technologies).

- Addressing the **social, economic and environmental determinants** of health as a means of reducing health inequities within and between countries.[54]

As far as they go, these are a reasonable set of priorities, but they fail to identify what would actually be the WHO's leadership role in respect of other actors both within and outside the health sector. The longer explanation of these leadership priorities and the WHO's role in the GPW provides little further guidance on exactly what the WHO will do.

The WHO should not be involved at country level in small technical assistance projects of no strategic importance that could or should be done by countries themselves, with or without the support of donors.

The working group considered that the distinction between 'core' and 'supportive' is not dissimilar to the distinction drawn between the WHO's normative functions (essentially standard-setting) and its technical assistance functions, as referred to in Chapter 1. On the other hand, 'core' functions in this framework are not necessarily normative and include elements of technical assistance. Thus some of the work for which the WHO is best known – such as its role in the elimination of smallpox, or in fighting pandemics and emerging diseases, or in research and development – involve activities and technical assistance that could not be described as normative but that are concerned with the delivery of global public goods. Equating the WHO's core work with its standard-setting role would therefore unduly circumscribe the range of activities that it should legitimately pursue. By the same token, equating all its technical assistance as 'supportive', and thus potentially better undertaken by another body or countries themselves when able to do so, would limit the WHO's ability both to provide global public goods and to support countries in the implementation of the guidelines, standards and agreements developed by the organization in its normative role.

These issues are discussed more fully in the following chapters, but the essence of the problem is that the WHO and its member states need to define more clearly the boundaries of the WHO's 'supportive' role, which should be related to its 'core' functions as a provider of global public goods. Thus it *should not be* involved at country level in small technical assistance projects of no strategic importance that could or *should be* done by countries themselves, with or without the support of donors. The WHO should be involved at country level in providing strategic advice relating to the implementation of its normative work, in monitoring the health situation and assessing health trends, in helping countries to implement international agreements such as the IHR and the FCTC, and in other matters that relate to the WHO's core functions and global health security as defined above.

---

[54] Proposed Programme Budget 2014–2015, A66/7, 19 April 2013, http://apps.who.int/gb/ebwha/pdf_files/WHA66/A66_7-en.pdf.

The other aspect requiring attention is the WHO's first function: *providing leadership on matters critical to health and engaging in partnerships where joint action is needed. As noted, the role of the WHO is not well defined in the current reform documentation.*[55]

The key difficulty in actually achieving this more focused approach on the part of the WHO relates to the kind of funding provided to the organization, discussed in Chapter 5, and the WHO's human resource profile.

The 2013 evaluation noted that:

> questions are now raised by Member States, Secretariat staff and NGOs as to whether the most appropriate capacity is in place to deliver concurrently on its historical areas of activity and on leadership priorities. The changing Member States needs will require staff to have more than scientific skills, e.g. economics, diplomatic and strategy-making. While re-profiling has happened in certain countries (e.g. Thailand, India), it has not been done at an organisation-wide level. The GPW does not address this important dimension.[55]

The WHO's professional staff are predominantly either health professionals or administrators. According to the latest annual human resources report,[56] nearly 48 per cent of staff fall in the former category, of whom more than 90 per cent are 'medical specialists'. Nearly 35 per cent are administrative specialists. Of the remainder, 1.6 per cent are social scientists, 1.4 per cent lawyers, 0.9 per cent environmental scientists and just 0.1 per cent economists. It is notable that in 2001 the administrative complement was only 26 per cent of all staff. Given the leadership priorities expressed by the WHO, it would seem apparent that this distribution of staff skills is sub-optimal. Addressing the social, economic and environmental determinants of health and non-communicable disease, and advising countries on the attainment of universal health coverage and financial protection would seem to demand a very different distribution of skills to that which exists currently.

In that context, it would be useful to think of two kinds of technical department in the WHO, requiring different skill mixes. One set of technical departments would be those with a traditional disease or medical focus, where a bias in favour of medical professionals may well be appropriate. Another set of departments might be focused on subject areas requiring both health and other kinds of expertise, such as departments dealing with social and economic determinants, statistics, health system financing and so on.

Moreover, the WHO has a very rapid staff turnover. In the next 10 years nearly 42 per cent of the WHO's professional staff will retire; and, typically, because many staff join in mid-career, 40–50 per cent of WHO staff retire in any 10-year period. Thus there is every opportunity for the WHO to adjust the composition of its professional staff over a relatively short period of time in order to reflect more closely its functions and leadership priorities.

Conclusions and proposals

The WHO has a dual role as a provider of global public goods that benefit all nations – rich and poor – and that need to be provided collectively, and as a provider of supportive services to its member states. The WHO's current definition of its core functions provides a sound basis, but given their level of generality these may not capture explicitly certain functions that are important, or may implicitly include functions that are less important.

Furthermore, the nature of the WHO's leadership role is largely undefined in the current core functions. This is with regard to both the health sector and relationships with governmental and non-governmental actors, and regarding decisions and actions outside the health sector that have an impact on health.

Recommendation 1: The WHO's core functions should provide explicitly for its work in promoting and maintaining global health security.

Recommendation 2: The WHO should provide strategic technical assistance to countries in support of its mission as a provider of global public goods. It should not seek to undertake activities that could or should be done better by others – by the host government with or without support from other agencies.

Recommendation 3: The WHO should undertake a review of the skill mix of its staff to ensure that it fits with its core functions and leadership priorities. Because the WHO has a rapid turnover of staff, significant changes could be made in a relatively short period.

---

[55] Second Stage Evaluation on WHO Reform.
[56] Human Resources: Annual Report, A66/36, 14 May 2013, http://apps.who.int/gb/ebwha/pdf_files/WHA66/A66_36-en.pdf.

3. Governance of the WHO: The Global Role

Introduction

One of the three planks of the internal reform programme is improved governance: focusing on improving the work of the governing bodies, including strengthening global–regional linkages. This is designed to foster a more strategic and disciplined approach to priority-setting, to enhance the oversight of the programmatic and financial aspects of the organization, and to improve the efficiency and inclusivity of intergovernmental consensus-building. The main components include strengthening the oversight function of the WHO governing bodies at global and regional levels; harmonizing and aligning governance processes at all levels; achieving more efficient decision-making by governing bodies; and agreeing on a framework for the engagement of the WHO with NGOs and the private sector.

The 2013 evaluation of the internal reform programme says that the WHO is making 'marginal progress' in improving governance – in terms of handling governing body meetings more effectively and being more strategic in decision-making.[57] While noting that there have been some 'quick wins' relating to procedure (e.g. a 'traffic light' system to limit speaking time), it emphasizes reluctance on the part of member states to accept any self-discipline for the sake of the greater good – i.e. more focus, fewer items, better discussion and better decisions. It suggests that the revised internal governance arrangements will be insufficient to modify this counterproductive member-state behaviour.

Among other things, it notes the lack of impact hitherto of the effort to reduce the number of agenda items at governing body meetings. Ironically, at the January 2014 EB at which the evaluation was presented, the director-general noted that there were '67 items on its agenda, with 17 resolutions […] by far the highest number of items ever scheduled for a non-budget year'.[58] Each resolution at the EB and the WHA is accompanied by an estimate from the Secretariat of the costs of implementation; whether or not this is provided for in the programme budget; and, if not or not wholly, what the funding gap is. Hitherto these estimates have been largely ignored by the EB and the WHA. However, the report from the January 2014 EB noted that it had 'adopted 20 resolutions, 14 recommending draft resolutions to the Health Assembly for consideration or adoption, and six decisions with cost implications. The projected costs to the Secretariat for the biennium 2014–2015 were US\$ 202.1 million, of which US\$ 37.8 million were not included in the Programme budget 2014–2015', and recommended that such a tabulation of the costs of draft resolutions be presented in future in advance of governing body meetings.[59]

In relation to the WHO's engagement with external stakeholders, the internal reform programme is exploring ways to collaborate more effectively with relevant stakeholders – including NGOs, partnerships, the private sector and foundations – with a view to promoting greater coherence in global health. The challenge, as seen by the WHO, is to determine how the WHO can engage with a wider range of players without undermining its intergovernmental nature or opening itself to influence by those with vested interests. Moreover, governance reforms aim to strengthen the multilateral role of the WHO and to capitalize more effectively on the WHO's leadership position in global health.

The 2013 evaluation notes the scant progress that has been achieved either in improving engagement with non-state actors or in strengthening the WHO's role in global health. In that context, the WHO has not yet effectively addressed what should be the right balance between its norm-setting and technical support roles.

The working group considered several times the roles that the WHO needs to perform in the light of the discussion in Chapter 2, and what this should mean for the structure of the organization itself and its governance. Underlying this consideration was, on the one hand, a desire to protect the integrity of the WHO's normative and technical work (particularly from political and commercial pressures) and, on the other hand, and somewhat in conflict, a desire that the WHO should be a vehicle for 'evidence-based participatory public policy-making' involving a range of stakeholders in that process. Thus one proposal was that there should be a public health institute, separate from the WHO, that would somehow be protected from political and commercial pressures. A further proposal was that the institute should be the platform for evidence-based participatory policy processes, thereby explicitly engaging with external stakeholders and their diverse interests and agendas. Beyond that, opinion was divided between those who thought that establishing a public health institute separate from the WHO would undermine and diminish the organization and that the objective should be achieved by an internal reform of the WHO, and those who thought that the WHO in its current form was simply incapable of undertaking such a task.

---

[57] Second Stage Evaluation on WHO Reform.

[58] Report by the Director-General to the Executive Board at its 134th session, EB134/2, 20 January 2014, http://apps.who.int/gb/ebwha/pdf_files/EB134/B134_2-en.pdf.

[59] Report of the Executive Board on its 133rd and 134th sessions, A67/2, 25 April 2014, http://apps.who.int/gb/ebwha/pdf_files/WHA67/A67_2-en.pdf.

Internal governance

Separating the political and the technical

The tension between the political and the technical has been around since the WHO's beginnings. The constitution specifies that a member of the EB should be 'a person technically qualified in the field of health'. The expectation of many at the time, including that of Brock Chisholm, the first director-general, was that such persons would sit in their personal capacity and, although nominated by member governments, would not act as government representatives. For Chisholm that was:

> [...] the greatest possible threat to the integrity of the Organization [...] the Assembly should be able to feel complete confidence that the advice it received from the Executive Board is based on technical considerations, and is entirely free of national or group interests of any kind or degree. Nothing short of complete world-mindedness is acceptable in any member of the Executive Board.[60]

In reality, this was always something of a fiction. In 1998 the WHA clarified that member states should designate their EB members as government representatives, technically qualified in the field of health.[61]

The working group was presented with a stimulating analysis of these issues, as part of which one proposal was to split the WHO into two.[62] This analysis contends that the WHO's functions as an independent technical authority on public health and as a platform for 'political' negotiations between governments have become inextricably entwined, to the detriment of the organization's effectiveness. The intrusion of the political into the technical undermines the latter by diluting the WHO's ability to issue fearless and independent advice on public health. The lack of emphasis on political secretariat functions, and the different skill mix this might require in the organization, undermines progress in the difficult political negotiations in the WHO's governing bodies. Therefore, separating the political and technical parts of the WHO could provide a solution.

This analysis attempts to make a clear distinction between the WHO's role as a neutral and objective 'non-political' technical agency, providing standards and guidelines and related technical support to countries; and its function as a deliberative body, bringing together governments to reach 'political' agreements as in a WHA resolution or a convention such as the FCTC. But this may overestimate the extent to which the technical can be separated from

the political. What makes WHO staff nervous of providing unbiased technical advice (for instance, about the burden of disease in a particular country) is the prospect of upsetting one or other member state by revealing unpalatable facts, evidence or conclusions. The fate of the WHO's work on the global burden of disease – established at the WHO during Gro Harlem Brundtland's tenure as director-general but now undertaken by the Institute of Health Metrics and Evaluation (IHME), financed principally by the Bill & Melinda Gates Foundation – is a good example of how potentially politically contentious work of critical public health importance was effectively deemed too hot to handle by the WHO when Brundtland departed. Nevertheless, the WHO is extremely defensive about the fact that it let this work go. The statement issued when the IHME issued its 2012 report on the global burden of disease is very revealing about the WHO's ambivalence on the subject, and concerning the difficulty of carrying out such technical work in a body 'accountable to Member States' without the freedoms that an academic environment allows.[63]

This kind of 'politicization' of technical work occurs independent of the fact that the WHO is also a policy-making body capable of negotiating international agreements on matters relating to public health. Therefore, splitting the WHO into two – between 'non-political' technical work and its policy-making role – does not resolve the adverse impact of 'politicization' while the WHO remains an intergovernmental body. The analogy is with national bodies such as the US Centers for Disease Control and Prevention (CDC) or the UK National Institute for Health and Care Excellence (NICE) – bodies set up with a specific technical mandate by national legislation that protects them (to a greater or lesser extent), subject to the rule of law, from direct political interference, although hardly from political controversy or indirect political influence.

But in an international organization context, such protections, legal or otherwise, cannot be easily replicated. There is no equivalent institutional structure in the international arena that can provide comparable shelter from interference by national governments. This is the difficulty, for instance, with the idea that a global public health institute could somehow be isolated from the political pressures that the WHO experiences. What form of governance could be defined to achieve that? A very good example is in the WHO constitution itself, which pledges every member state 'to respect the exclusively international

[60] Quoted in Farley, J., *Brock Chisholm, the World Health Organization, and the Cold War* (Vancouver, BC: UBC Press, 2008), pp. 69–70.
[61] Review of the Constitution and Regional Arrangements of the World Health Organization. Status of Members of the Executive Board. Clarification of the Interpretation of Article 24 of the WHO Constitution, WHA51.26, 16 May 1998, http://apps.who.int/iris/bitstream/10665/79878/1/ear26.pdf?ua=1.
[62] Hoffman, J. and Røttingen, J.-A., 'Split WHO in Two: Strengthening Political Decision-making and Securing Independent Advice', *Public Health* 128 (2014): 188–94, http://download.journals.elsevierhealth.com/pdfs/journals/0033-3506/PIIS0033350613002916.pdf.
[63] *Global Burden of Disease 2010 Study*, 13 December 2012, http://www.who.int/mediacentre/news/statements/2012/global_burden_disease_20121213/en/index.html.

character of the Director-General and the staff and not to seek to influence them'. Is there any nation that has respected this injunction? Rather the opposite: national delegations in Geneva are there principally for that purpose.

Nevertheless, the problem highlighted in this analysis is a real one. The WHO is hampered in its technical work by the need to accommodate, as best it can, the preferences, policies, and political and economic interests of member states – even where these may conflict with public health advice. Margaret Chan has herself noted:

> Market power readily translates into political power. Few governments prioritize health over big business [...] Not one single country has managed to turn around its obesity epidemic in all age groups. This is not a failure of individual will-power. This is a failure of political will to take on big business [...] When industry is involved in policy-making, rest assured that the most effective control measures will be downplayed or left out entirely. This, too, is well documented, and dangerous. In the view of WHO, the formulation of health policies must be protected from distortion by commercial or vested interests.[64]

In 1948 tobacco was not on the WHO's agenda. The first two official histories of the WHO (covering the period up to 1968) do not mention smoking or tobacco. Yet the first definitive evidence on the harmful effects of smoking appeared in the 1950s and the famous report to the US Surgeon-General in 1964 persuasively set out all the available evidence.[65] The first, quite tentative, resolution at the WHA on the harmful effects of smoking did not appear until 1970.[66] And it was not until 1987 that smoking was banned on WHO premises – with the symbolic smashing of an ashtray by the then Director-General, Halfdan Mahler.[67] Only in 1998, under Brundtland, did the WHO establish the Tobacco Free Initiative, which ultimately led to agreement on the FCTC in 2003 and its entry into force in 2005. How many lives might have been saved if the WHO had adopted a more determined approach from the beginning?

There is no easy way to deal with these political realities, but the example of tobacco shows that determined leadership, as demonstrated by Brundtland, is an essential prerequisite if opposition from commercial interests and governments motivated by commercial objectives is to be overcome.

Apart from determined leadership, there may be other ways to limit political interference. One proposal is that rather than splitting the WHO into two, it should be reorganized internally between technical departments and those

dealing with governance and management. This could be done by creating two posts of deputy director-general to replace the existing single post. One would be responsible for the WHO's technical departments, but importantly would also have the status of chief scientist with specific responsibility for ensuring the quality and integrity of the WHO's evidence-based technical work in its six technical clusters. The other, equivalent to a chief operating officer, would be responsible for the General Management Cluster and, as appropriate, other functions currently undertaken in the director-general's office such as preparations for negotiations at the WHA. This would provide an internal structure that assigns clear responsibility at a senior level for the technical functions of the WHO on the one hand, and its policy-making and managerial functions on the other, divided between the director-general and the chief operating officer. In this context, it should be noted that the 2012 JIU report stated that the role of the current deputy director-general was ill-defined and that there would be benefit in assigning this role specific responsibilities, thereby freeing the director-general to concentrate on strategic and global issues.

Electing the director-general

An obvious aspect of the political process in the WHO is the election of the director-general. The constitution does not provide any guidance on term limits for the director-general, or for RDs. The second director-general, Marcel Candau, served for 20 years (1953–73) and the third, Halfdan Mahler, for 15 years (1973–88). Some RDs have served even longer: for example, Hussein A. Gezairy served 30 years as RD of the Eastern Mediterranean Regional Office (EMRO) in 1982–2012.

Unlimited possibilities for re-election increase the extent to which political considerations, and the quest for re-election, influence the behaviour of directors-general and of RDs throughout their tenure. This applies in particular to the way in which the resources under their control, and the influence they are able to exert (e.g. through making appointments), are utilized to further their electoral prospects. There is clearly therefore a potential conflict with the duties of impartiality and integrity that the constitution enjoins on its officers (and its member states). Apart from considerations of encouraging politicization of the WHO, extreme longevity of leadership is undesirable in almost any organization. The 1993 Executive Board Working Group on the WHO

---

[64] Opening address at the 8th Global Conference on Health Promotion, Helsinki, Finland, 10 June 2013, http://www.who.int/dg/speeches/2013/health_promotion_20130610/en/index.html.

[65] *Smoking and Health: Report of the Advisory Committee to the Surgeon General of the Public Health Service* (Washington, DC: US Government Printing Office, 1964), http://profiles.nlm.nih.gov/NN/B/B/M/Q/_/nnbbmq.pdf.

[66] Health Consequences of Smoking, WHA23.32, May 1970, http://www.who.int/tobacco/framework/wha_eb/wha23_32/en/.

[67] 'Guardians of world's health find it hard to quit smoking', *New York Times*, 19 May 1987, http://www.nytimes.com/1987/05/19/world/guardians-of-world-s-health-find-it-hard-to-quit-smoking.html.

Response to Global Change cited the 'growing complexity and demands placed on the highest executive leadership of WHO, and [...] the availability of highly capable health professionals within and outside the Organization' as reasons for limiting the number of terms for the director-general and RDs, or for increasing the duration of a term but restricting the office-holder to one term.[68] It is significant, and no doubt not unrelated, that these conclusions followed closely on the controversies concerning Hiroshi Nakajima's re-election in 1993 (referred to in Chapter 1).

Accordingly, in 1996 the WHA agreed to limit the director-general to one five-year term, renewable once, but existing incumbents were exempted.[69] In 1998 the EB extended the same rule to RDs, with the same exemption.[70] Thus Gezairy was able to remain in post for a further 14 years, until 2012.

The WHO has not been very successful in developing a broader interface with civil society and other non-governmental groups. A number of NGOs and some member states are inherently suspicious of the private sector's motives for collaborating with the WHO.

The desirability of bolstering the independence and autonomy of the director-general as much as possible, and of minimizing the intrusion of political factors, suggests that there is merit in extending this principle on the lines suggested by the 1993 EB Working Group by allowing the director-general to serve only one term, but of seven years.

A further proposal considered was for the director-general to be elected by an open rather than secret ballot. This could be a partial safeguard against country delegates being subjected to, or succumbing to, vote-buying practices of one kind or another. However, because the concept of the secret ballot is so ingrained in international consciousness as the cornerstone of democracy, and because it is universal within the UN system in electing organization heads, it is hard to see such a reform being successfully adopted. It is important, nevertheless, to recognize that the process of electing a WHO director-general is very different from that involved in electing a candidate or a president in a national election. The voters in the former case should be executing a deliberate decision made by their government in favour of one or other candidate. An open ballot might prevent pressure being exerted on the delegate who actually casts the vote, but not, of course, pressure or inducements that might have been brought to bear to influence the government's decision on whom to vote for.

Governance of and for health

More than in almost all other UN institutions, member states in the WHO resist the direct involvement of non-state actors in policy-making processes. But, as the 'directing and co-ordinating' authority, it is to be expected that the WHO would play a role in providing a platform or mechanism for these numerous actors to exchange views and information and to coordinate their efforts better. But the dilemma in the internal reform programme is described by senior WHO officials as follows:

> [...] whatever form coordination takes, it requires that WHO engage effectively with a much wider range of stakeholders – from different parts of governments, civil society, the private sector and other non-state actors – than was the case in 1948. Without such engagement, it is unlikely that coordination at global or national level will be effective. But therein lies the challenge for an inter-governmental organization in a multistakeholder world. How to secure meaningful engagement on one hand, whilst ensuring, to the satisfaction of a critical audience, that WHO's normative role is fully safeguarded from vested interests, and that the prerogative of governments to have an exclusive role in decision making is preserved?[71]

Some institutions have been created particularly to promote coordination between the biggest funders of global health. For example, the International Health Partnership, founded in 2007, is a group of international organizations, foundations, bilateral agencies and country governments working together to put internationally agreed principles for effective health aid and development cooperation into practice. It is a joint enterprise between the WHO and the World Bank. Another initiative, also established in 2007, was the Health 8 (H8), an informal group of the WHO, UNICEF, the UN Population Fund (UNFPA), UNAIDS, the Global Fund, GAVI, the Bill & Melinda Gates Foundation and the World Bank, seeking to coordinate action around achieving the MDGs. However, this seems to be currently inactive: the 2013 evaluation proposes that it should be revived and its role enhanced. In general, the evaluation found that the WHO and its member states had not yet seriously addressed the organization's wider role in global health governance.

Apart from the contacts with civil society and academia on specific and professionally defined issues, the WHO has not been very successful in developing a broader interface with civil society and other non-governmental groups. A

---

[68] Report of the Executive Board Working Group on WHO Response to Global Change, EB92/4, 16 April 1993, http://hist.library.paho.org/English/GOV/CD/15660.pdf.
[69] WHO Reform and Response to Global Change: Report of the Ad Hoc Group, WHA49.7, 23 May 1996, http://hist.library.paho.org/English/GOV/CD/15660.pdf.
[70] Amendments to Rules of Procedure of the Executive Board: Term of Office of Regional Directors, EB102.R1, 18 May 1998.
[71] Cassells, A. et al., 'Reforming WHO: The Art of the Possible', *Public Health* 128 (2014): 2, http://download.journals.elsevierhealth.com/pdfs/journals/0033-3506/PIIS0033350613004034.pdf.

number of NGOs and some member states are inherently suspicious of the private sector's motives for collaborating with the WHO. It is this context that reinforces the WHO Secretariat's excessive caution about deepening relationships with both the private sector and NGOs in the face of this mutual hostility.

One idea promoted by the Secretariat was the World Health Forum, a body including all non-governmental stakeholders which would meet periodically. As seen by the WHO, its purpose would be 'to explore, in an informal and multi-stakeholder setting, ways in which the major actors in global health can work more effectively together – globally and at country level – to increase effectiveness, coherence and accountability and to reduce fragmentation and duplication of effort.'[72] But this idea did not prove attractive to many member states, or to the NGO community itself. They were not convinced about its added value, and had many questions about its representativeness and inclusiveness, and how it would address conflicts of interest and not infringe on the sovereignty of the WHO's existing governance bodies. As a result, the proposal was formally dropped. An earlier proposal on similar lines was for a committee C at the WHA, where non-state actors could be involved in deliberations and make recommendations for inclusion in decisions by the intergovernmental committees A and B.[73] This proposal too has made no headway.

The evaluation notes that the role that the WHO should play in the global health architecture has not been discussed in detail either by member states or by the Secretariat. When a paper on this subject was submitted to the EB in January 2013,[74] it was considered only briefly and further discussion was deferred to the next EB. At that EB in May 2013, discussion on the successor paper, which dealt with relations with non-state actors and the WHO's role in global health governance, resulted in a decision, suggested by the Secretariat, that ignored any comment on the latter issue but requested further work in relation to non-state actors.[75] Accordingly, at the January 2014 EB there was further development of the work on non-state actors but no reference to the WHO's role in global health governance. A member state consultation on the WHO's proposals for engagement with non-state actors[76] in March 2014, however, seems only to have confirmed existing divisions between member states, particularly with regard to differentiating between those NGOs that represent industry interests, and others.

In relation to global health governance, the May 2013 EB paper had noted:

> The 'seat' of global health governance is becoming more diverse. In other words, decisions that influence global health governance are being made in a growing number of arenas. In particular, health issues are beginning to feature prominently on the agenda of the United Nations General Assembly, notably in relation to universal health coverage and noncommunicable diseases. The number and range of decision-making bodies, globally and regionally, requires that WHO make careful strategic choices as to where it can most effectively influence outcomes.[77]

This is not the voice of an organization that is confident of the role it should play as a 'coordinator' of global health work. Nor does it seek to define, even if it does not see a central role for the WHO, what those 'careful strategic choices' might be. The fact is that member states also, as in fact the quotation illustrates, give no indication that they see the WHO as the linchpin of all global health work. But nor are they providing any coherent guidance to the WHO as to where it can make a bigger contribution in line with its unique position as the only universal intergovernmental institution in global health. As the 2013 evaluation put it:

> Member States are increasingly expecting WHO to be at the centre of the coordination with the UN family and other development partners on health matters. Some Member States have mentioned the need for WHO to collaborate in a more active manner with regional groupings (e.g. UNASUR, ASEAN). [WHO's] approach comes across as still inward-looking in nature, with the risk of having a less integrated WHO with decreased leveraging power and authority. WHO's current operating model does not provide confidence that the organisation will be capable to deliver against its expectations. A more robust articulation of how WHO will set out to deliver on [its] objectives, notably the alignment of country offices with country's needs, the definition of mechanisms for coordination across the levels and geographies of the organization and a better definition of WHO's strategic approach to partnering with stakeholders will position the Organization to be more effective.[78]

The working group discussed these issues intensely but it was also unable to come up with new strategies for a global approach to interaction with stakeholders, given the history of initiatives in this area to date. The essential problem is that proposals such as those for a World Health Forum are mechanisms looking for a *raison d'être*. Since mistrust exists between some of the parties involved, proposals with no specific objectives or problems to tackle – beyond considering how the major actors in global health can work more effectively together – provide no basis for overcoming them.

[72] World Health Forum, Concept Paper, 22 June 2011, http://www.who.int/dg/reform/en_who_reform_world_health_forum.pdf.
[73] Silberschmidt, G., Matheson, D. and Kickbusch, I., 'Creating a Committee C of the World Health Assembly', *The Lancet* (2008), Vol. 371: 1483–86, http://graduateinstitute.ch/files/live/sites/iheid/files/sites/globalhealth/shared/1894/Article%20Committee%20C%20The%20Lancet%203%20May%2008.pdf.
[74] WHO's Role in Global Health Governance, EB132/5 Add5, 18 January 2013, http://apps.who.int/gb/ebwha/pdf_files/EB132/B132_5Add5-en.pdf.
[75] EB133 (2) WHO Governance Reform, 29 May 2013, http://apps.who.int/gb/ebwha/pdf_files/EB133/B133_DIV2-en.pdf.
[76] Background document to support discussion of WHO's engagement with non-state actors, 20 March 2014, http://www.who.int/about/who_reform/background-non_state_actors_en.pdf?ua=1.
[77] WHO Governance Reform. EB133/16, 17 May 2013, http://apps.who.int/gb/ebwha/pdf_files/EB133/B133_16-en.pdf.
[78] Second Stage Evaluation on WHO Reform.

That is why others, such as the Lancet-University of Oslo Commission cited in Chapter 1, have suggested that the WHO should not play a central role in global health governance ('governance for health'). Figure 2 reproduces its concept of a platform that might integrate a wide range of governments, non-state actors and agencies in monitoring the health effects of policies pursued in other sectors that may have an impact on health. The WHO is presented as peripheral to this, but central to governance in the health sector ('governance of health'). At the same time, how such a platform – much more complex than envisaged in the WHO's World Health Forum proposal – could be constructed and governed, and indeed under whose aegis it should be located, was raised as an issue but not answered in the report. Nor was a solution given as to how the problems encountered by the WHO in establishing a similar platform could be overcome in this new setting.

However, the working group noted that the more successful examples of cooperation between the WHO and external stakeholders occurred around specific issues. For example, the WHO Pandemic Influenza Preparedness

Framework, agreed in 2011, brings the WHO together with member states, industry and other stakeholders to implement a global approach to pandemic influenza preparedness and response; it is widely regarded as a significant step forward, including industry contributions towards running the system.[79] The Prequalification Programme, established in 2001, is a service tailored to the needs of UN and other agencies to facilitate access to medicines that meet unified standards of quality, safety and efficacy, and has played a significant role in facilitating global access to quality medicines by working with industry and regulatory authorities in the developed and developing worlds.[80] The WHO's work on neglected tropical diseases has long involved partnerships with pharmaceutical companies that donate medicines, and with governments and NGOs involved in their distribution.[81] The WHO also has a long-standing partnership with Health Action International on medicine prices and availability that has undertaken pioneering work on data collection and evidence gathering; and, more recently, a partnership on policy proposals to be derived from that evidence.[82]

Figure 2: Multi-stakeholder platform on governance for health

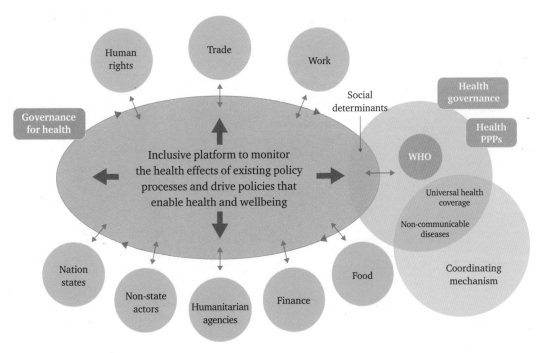

Source: Lancet-Oslo Commission © The Lancet/University of Oslo.

---

[79] Pandemic Influenza Preparedness (PIP) Framework, http://www.who.int/influenza/pip/en/.
[80] Prequalification Programme. A United Nations Programme Managed by WHO, http://apps.who.int/prequal/default.htm.
[81] Neglected Tropical Diseases, WHA66.12, 27 May 2013, http://apps.who.int/gb/ebwha/pdf_files/WHA66/A66_R12-en.pdf.
[82] WHO/Health Action International Project on Medicine Prices and Availability, http://www.who.int/medicines/areas/access/Medicine_Prices_and_Availability/en/.

Conclusions and proposals

The WHO is both a technical agency and a policy-making body. The excessive intrusion of political considerations in its technical work can damage its authority and credibility as a standard-bearer for health. Determined leadership is necessary to overcome political and economic interests that threaten public health goals. But politics cannot realistically be wholly separated from the WHO's technical work.

Apart from leadership, there are two proposals that may reduce the harmful effects of politicization. One proposal is not to divide the WHO into two, but to separate more clearly its technical and policy-making roles. The second is to further limit the term of the director-general.

Recommendation 4: The WHO should provide an internal separation between the WHO's technical departments and those dealing with governance and management by creating two posts of deputy director-general, with one to be responsible for each.

Recommendation 5: The WHO should allow the director-general a single, seven-year term, without the possibility of re-election.

The WHO's plans for greater involvement of non-governmental stakeholders in its processes seem to have reached a dead end. The observation of the working group was that collaboration with these stakeholders has been most successful where it is built around tackling a specific task or problem where mutual confidence and trust can be built through constructive endeavour.

Recommendation 6: The WHO should explore new avenues for collaboration with non-governmental actors that have a concrete and specific purpose.

4. Governance of the WHO: Regions and Countries

Introduction

The WHO is a large and highly decentralized organization, with more than 7,000 employees on its staff and more than 150 offices worldwide – including the headquarters and six regional offices. Its distinctive feature, unique among international organizations, is the independent governance structure for each of its six regional offices. About three-quarters of staff work in the regional and country offices, which account for about 65 per cent of total expenditure (Figure 3). In addition the WHO employs, according to its annual human resources report, over 3,000 staff (full-time equivalent) on non-staff contracts although it is not clear how this is reconciled with the over 6,000 non-staff contracts under the Global Polio Eradication Initiative.[83]

The WHO's distinctive feature is the independent governance structure for each of its six regional offices. About three-quarters of staff work in the regional and country offices, which account for about 65 per cent of total expenditure.

Despite this fact, however, the internal reform programme has not devoted any significant attention to considering whether this distribution of WHO resources makes sense in terms of the functions that the WHO needs to perform, or whether this configuration is the most cost-effective way to deliver those functions. Rather, the status quo is broadly taken as a parameter, allowing the possibility of only incremental change to the existing structure.

Figure 3: Staffing and expenditure, by offices

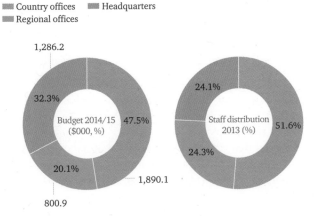

■ Country offices ■ Headquarters
■ Regional offices

Sources: Proposed Programme Budget 2014–2015, A66/7, 19 April 2013, http://apps.who.int/gb/ebwha/pdf_files/WHA66/A66_7-en.pdf. Human Resources: Annual Report, A67/47, 17 April 2014.

The regions

The WHO has six regional offices:

- Africa (AFRO), based in Brazzaville
- Americas (AMRO/PAHO), based in Washington DC
- South-East Asia (SEARO), based in New Delhi
- Europe (EURO), based in Copenhagen
- Eastern Mediterranean (EMRO), based in Cairo
- Western Pacific (WPRO), based in Manila

History of the WHO's regional structure

The WHO's regional structure cannot be understood without knowing its history. In the post-war discussions about its establishment, the most controversial issue was whether existing regional organizations, of which the Pan American Sanitary Bureau (PASB) was the most important example, should be an integral part of the WHO or remain as autonomous institutions but with close links to WHO headquarters. The PASB (initially called the International Sanitary Bureau) was established in 1902, hosted by the US Public Health Service. Later renamed the Pan American Sanitary Organization (PASO), this was the origin of what is now the Pan American Health Organization (PAHO). Politics, as well as ideology, played a key part in this controversy.

One group (including the Norwegian, British and Canadian representatives) favoured regional organizations, but only as integral parts of the global organization. Another group, led by the US and French representatives, believed that autonomous regional organizations (notably the PASB) could exist alongside the WHO and its own regional organizations. In fact, the second group was in some respects positively hostile to the whole idea of the WHO. The first group believed that an autonomous regional organization would weaken the WHO and that there should be one, single organization.[84]

Key points of the compromise reached in the constitution as agreed were:

- Regional organizations would be integral parts of the WHO;
- Each would have a regional committee, composed of member states, with its own rules of procedure and a regional office to execute its decisions;

---

[83] Table 13 in Annex 1 of Human Resources: Annual Report. A67/47, 17 April 2014, http://www.who.int/about/resources_planning/Annex_A67_47-en.pdf?ua=1 for lower number. Annex to Human Resources: Annual Report, A67/47, 17 April 2014, http://apps.who.int/gb/ebwha/pdf_files/WHA67/A67_47-en.pdf for polio number.
[84] Farley, *Brock Chisholm, the World Health Organization, and the Cold War.*

- The head of the regional office would be the RD, appointed by the EB in agreement with the regional committee; and

- The staff of the regional office would be appointed in a manner to be determined by agreement between the director-general and the RD.

The constitution also specified, in Article 54, that PASO and all other intergovernmental regional health organizations in existence would in due course be integrated with the WHO. This 'would be effected as soon as practicable through common action based on mutual consent of the competent authorities expressed through the organizations concerned'. As it was, agreement was reached in 1949 whereby PASO would serve as the Regional Office of the WHO and its existing governing body as the regional committee. But the agreement confirmed that each organization would also retain its own name and identity, and that PASO could promote its own programmes in the Americas provided these were compatible with the WHO's policy and programmes and were separately financed.[85]

In effect, PASO had won the battle for 'decentralization'. The autonomous status of PASO was further emphasized when it shortly after became a specialized agency of the Organization of American States (OAS). As the first WHO Director-General, Brock Chisholm, noted, it was impossible to serve two masters.[86] Thus the injunction in the WHO constitution for 'integration in due course' effectively became a dead letter. In 1995 a report to the EB noted 'that in the light of the expectation of integration of PAHO and the WHO, which had not been fully accomplished in 50 years, the Organization should examine with PAHO whether (a) the Article should be amended or deleted, or (b) integration should be completed'.[87] Needless to say, no such examination has taken place.

PASO was therefore the model that determined the structure of the WHO's other regional organizations. These adopted a similar governance structure to PASO's, with regional committees of member states as the governing bodies and an RD elected by member states. Although the constitution provides for formal authority over the regional bodies to reside with the WHO's governing bodies and the director-general, the reality is that the latter have little real influence over the conduct or staffing of regional offices because *de facto* authority rests with the RD, elected by regional member states. However, unlike PASO, the other

regional offices are not in practice funded principally by direct contributions from member states in the region, but rather as part of the WHO's overall budget derived from member states as a whole, and from voluntary contributions and other sources of income available to the WHO.

Regional governance

As noted in Chapter 1, the regional question has continued to manifest itself in deliberations about WHO governance, and the tensions between the Geneva headquarters and regional offices are palpable in every discussion with WHO staff. The 1993 report by the JIU,[88] which considered the WHO's three-layer structure highly problematic, stressed that 'courageous reforms' (underlined in the original) were necessary if the WHO was to achieve its 'vast potential'. It identified the way in which RDs were elected by their regional committees as the central problem.

On the basis of that analysis, the JIU report suggested that the regional committees should be reviewed 'to ensure that they are more technically-oriented than politically-oriented'. In particular, it recommended that the director-general should, after consultation with the regional committees, select and nominate RDs for confirmation by the EB. The selection and consultation process should be confidential, and there should be no open competition (i.e. election) for the RD position. On this basis, it hoped that this would make RDs 'technical managers [...] fully involved, non-political, hands-on managers of their regional programmes'.

The JIU thought all this could be done without changing the constitution (elections of RDs or of the director-general are not referred to, only their appointment by the EB and WHA respectively). On the other hand, it is clear to see that, apart from any other consideration, a confidential process behind closed doors would not necessarily appear to be an improvement on the status quo in terms of transparency and accountability. For this among other reasons, it is unsurprising that the JIU recommendations were not followed up.

A further review by the JIU was commissioned as part of the current reform programme in 2012.[89] The JIU again examined the quality of governance at regional level. It concluded that there is 'little oversight of the work of regional offices by Regional Committees'. Very few management reports are provided to the committees, and

[85] World Health Organization, Basic Documents, 47th Edition. Agreements with Other Intergovernmental Organizations, http://apps.who.int/gb/bd/PDF/bd47/EN/agreements-with-other-inter-en.pdf.

[86] Farley, *Brock Chisholm, the World Health Organization, and the Cold War*.

[87] *WHO Reform: Review of the Constitution and Regional Arrangements of the World Health Organization. Report of the Special Group*, EB101/7, 14 November 1997, http://apps.who.int/gb/archive/pdf_files/EB101/pdfangl/eb1017.pdf.

[88] Joint Inspection Unit, 'Decentralization of Organizations within the United Nations System. Part III: The World Health Organization', Geneva, 1993, https://www.unjiu.org/en/reports-notes/JIU%20Products/JIU_REP_1993_2_ENGLISH.pdf.

[89] 'Review of Management, Administration and Decentralization in the World Health Organization' (see note 29).

those that are generate limited interest and action. The amount of information provided on management and programme budget implementation was somewhat better at AMRO/PAHO and EURO than at the other four offices, although even in these two there was little substantive discussion of that information, or decisions or resolutions providing guidance to the RD.

The JIU also conducted a staff survey assessing their opinion of various management issues in the WHO. By far the most striking finding was that, in the WHO overall, only 16 per cent of staff felt that the level of coordination and cooperation between headquarters and the regional offices was adequate, although an additional 44 per cent thought it 'somewhat adequate'. The most dissatisfaction was at headquarters, where one-third of staff thought the relationship inadequate.[90] A follow-up survey for the 2013 evaluation found that only 18 per cent in headquarters agreed that there was sufficient coordination, while 46 per cent disagreed.[91]

Nevertheless, the JIU, although concurring with its 1993 analysis, was prepared to accept the current director-general's view that the same objective could be achieved by better teamwork and creating a culture of 'One WHO' without changing his or her role in the selection process for RDs. This would involve increasing the role of the Global Policy Group (GPG – the consultative group of the director-general plus the six RDs) and strengthening the accountability of senior management. To that end, the JIU recommended reinforcing the role of the GPG by means of a formal resolution at the WHA institutionalizing its existence.

As noted in Chapter 1, the JIU recommendations were pushed back by the EB for the director-general to decide.

Regional composition

The 2012 JIU report also reviewed the composition of WHO regions. It noted the arbitrary delineation between the AFRO and EMRO regions, with several North African states included in EMRO rather than AFRO. Similarly, some countries are arbitrarily assigned to the SEARO and WPRO regions, while neighbouring countries (e.g. the two Koreas) are arbitrarily assigned to one or other of these regions. Moreover, the regions are very uneven in size in terms of the number of member states (although they are more balanced in terms of population). Thus AFRO has 46 members, but SEARO and WPRO together have 38 members. The JIU considered that 'having two Asian regional offices is not

fully justifiable on the basis of organizational, public health, or economic considerations'. In addition, it pointed out the lack of alignment with existing regional groupings of other UN organizations. In consequence, the JIU felt that a 'redefinition of the current regional design would enhance [the WHO's] operational cost-effectiveness'. Recognizing the issue was 'highly political', the report invited the director-general to consider ways to bring the issue to the attention of the WHA, which had the constitutional authority to modify geographical areas.

Working group analysis

The working group's own investigations confirmed this analysis – i.e. that the current WHO regions are a product of the immediate post-war area, and their configuration is heavily influenced by political criteria rather than by any considerations of shared health conditions and epidemiology. Furthermore, despite the possibility allowed for in the constitution, WHO regions have not evolved to accommodate new regional political organizations, many of which have health as part of their agenda. Thus EURO has remained essentially unchanged as the European Union has expanded to 28 member states, and in the context of the creation of many new countries as a result of the break-up of the Soviet Union. The 1993 JIU report also called for action to address the challenges of meeting the needs of 20 new members from the former Soviet bloc. Other regional entities that cut across WHO regions include the African Union (AU), the Association of Southeast Asian Nations (ASEAN) and the South Asian Association for Regional Cooperation (SAARC). The only region that can be considered to have a logical political basis is AMRO, which – as part of PAHO – is exactly aligned with the membership of the OAS. Although the WHO has also established subregional offices (e.g. within AMRO, AFRO and WPRO), these are not always aligned with subregional political entities. For example, the office for southern and eastern African countries, based in Harare (Zimbabwe), is mainly composed of the member countries of the Southern African Development Community (SADC), based in Gaborone (Botswana), but also covers countries as far afield as Eritrea, 2,400 miles away.

Different regional models

In the light of these findings, the working group considered a number of proposals for reforming the WHO's regional structure. Most of the group agreed that it needed to be

---

[90] Supplementary Paper to JIU/REP/2012/6&7: Review of Management, Administration and Decentralization in the World Health Organization (WHO). Analysis of the Results of WHO Staff Survey, Joint Inspection Unit. November 2012, https://www.unjiu.org/en/reports-notes/Other%20related%20documents/Suppl_Doc_Staff%20Survey%20analysis_15%20November%202012.pdf.
[91] WHO Evaluation Reform Staff Survey Analysis, PwC, October 2013, http://www.who.int/about/who_reform/whoreform-stage2evaluation-appen2-pwc-2013.pdf?ua=1.

reformed. The lack of consensus related to how it should be reformed and to the likelihood that member states would agree to any substantial change. Viewed pragmatically, moreover, the likely benefits of any proposed reform needed to be weighed against the costs of the upheaval that it would cause in the short term. But the group came back to discussing alternative models that reflected in large measure the debates at the time of the WHO's establishment. On the one hand, one could consider a unitary model ('One WHO'), as the opponents of PAHO/PASO autonomy had argued then; or, on the other, one could consider a decentralized model, as had prevailed in the case of PAHO.

A unitary model

A significant number of the working group supported the contention that abolition of the regional offices would not adversely affect the WHO's ability to carry out its functions and would in fact enhance it. Modern communications have significantly reduced the need for intermediary organizations between offices at country and headquarters level. Organizations such as the UK Department for International Development (DFID) and the World Bank have largely eliminated their regional offices. Abolition of the WHO regional offices would release significant financial and human resources that could be used more effectively in the WHO or elsewhere. It would centralize decision-making in Geneva and remove the tensions and inefficiencies inherent in the current, three-tiered structure. The WHO would then become, in governance terms, like other UN and international agencies, in deciding whether or not to establish regional and country offices according to what was needed to meet its objectives.

A decentralized model

An alternative approach would be to grasp the PAHO model whereby member states in a region are the principal funders of their regional organization. This would recognize that the value of regional offices should be tested by assessing the actual demand that countries have for a regional office. In its 2014/15 programme budget, PAHO projects that just over 70 per cent of its programmes will be financed by assessed and voluntary contributions from PAHO member states. The remainder of the budget is provided by the contribution from the WHO's assessed and voluntary contributions.[92] The WHO constitution actually notes that regional committees can 'recommend additional regional appropriations by the Governments of the respective regions if the proportion of the central budget of the Organization allotted to that region is insufficient for the carrying-out of the regional functions'.

This would allow the demand for regional services from the WHO to be 'market-tested'. The working group noted that although there were tensions between the WHO and PAHO, PAHO member states were firmly committed to its existence as an autonomous body, and its reputation for providing services that were valued by member states was, on the whole, higher than that of other regional offices. While the causative link could not be established definitively, the fact that member states were paying direct for this organization is a plausible reason for this. The 2012 JIU report noted that PAHO was:

> [...] ahead of the administrative and management practices of WHO headquarters and other regional offices. This has been possible thanks to the high degree of regional autonomy and decentralized decision-making, and to its healthy financial situation, which result from the will of its Member States to make assessed and voluntary contributions to both PAHO and WHO.[93]

There could be various ways to operationalize this decentralized model. Currently, approximately two-thirds of assessed contributions flow from Geneva to the regions. This flow could be capped at a lower level, or halted altogether, and member states (outside the Americas) could be asked to provide some or all of their assessed contribution to the WHO direct to the regional office as a substitute for subventions from Geneva.

Universalizing the PAHO model would institutionalize the decentralization of the WHO. It would make explicit that there were 'seven WHOs, not one'. The harmonization issues that give rise to continuing tensions between PAHO and the WHO would be compounded sixfold.

As it happens, the assessed contribution from the PAHO member states to the WHO is about 30 per cent of total assessed contributions; this is close to the amount of total assessed contributions actually retained by WHO headquarters (i.e. one-third) – the rest being distributed to the regions. Thus phasing out the annual 'subsidy' to the regions (including PAHO) would be at no net cost to headquarters or (unless they felt motivated to be more generous to the regional organizations than they currently are to the WHO as a whole) to member states. It would simply mean that funds would flow direct from member states to the regions and encourage member states to hold them more accountable than in the past.

---

[92] PAHO Program and Budget: 2014–2015. Off. Doc. 346 (Eng.), 1 September 2013, http://www.paho.org/hq/index.php?option=com_content&view=article&id=8833&Itemid=40033&lang=en#official.
[93] 'Review of Management, Administration and Decentralization in the World Health Organization'.

Because the WHO's overall operation is predominantly funded by voluntary, not assessed, contributions, the extent of this change should not be exaggerated. On the other hand, it would give cause to member states to think more carefully about the value of their regional office, and possibly consider whether there are other ways in which regional needs for health support could be met – including by considering strengthening the health agendas of existing regional organizations such as the AU or ASEAN.

The working group also noted that universalizing the PAHO model, if this is what might happen, would institutionalize the decentralization of the WHO. It would make explicit that there were 'seven WHOs, not one'. The harmonization issues that give rise to continuing tensions between PAHO and the WHO would be compounded sixfold. To the extent that happened, consideration might be given to reconfiguring the WHO so that regional offices, or other regional organizations, would have an explicit arm's-length relationship with the WHO and not be integral parts of the organization. Thus WHO headquarters would become 'the WHO', but the existing regional organizations would cease to be parts of it. Rather, the WHO would enter into partnerships with the regional organizations and/or others, exactly as it does now – for instance with the AU or ASEAN.

Country offices

Historical context

As previously noted, this issue has also been extensively debated in the past. A key finding of the donor-sponsored study[94] in 1997 was that the WHO needed to tailor its role to the needs of individual countries: there was a very poor or negative correlation between a country's needs and the scale of WHO efforts. In many countries with the least capacity, the WHO made a smaller contribution than in better-resourced countries. The study proposed the concept of 'essential presence', based on a thorough analysis of a country's current needs and capacities. If there was a need for a WHO presence, then a time-limited contract should be negotiated, defining the organization's role and responsibilities in relation to the government and other actors/donors. Such an arrangement should be regularly

reviewed, with a view to increasing a country's own responsibilities as its capacity increased.

The subsequent report to the EB,[95] which recommended radical change (as outlined in Chapter 1), was followed by a recommendation from the EB that the criteria for classifying countries should be further developed and that RDs 'should determine, in consultation with countries, whether the type of WHO representation in each country is appropriate, taking into account the Human Development Index and immunization coverage as indicators, and retaining the possibility of modifying representation in some countries'.[96] Little seems to have come of this decision, which occurred just before Gro Harlem Brundtland took office as director-general. A review by the new director-general in December 1999 devoted one small paragraph to the 'criteria for country presence', stating that these were currently being reviewed and additional criteria determined.[97]

The 2001 JIU report[98] recommended that priority be given to finalizing the work initiated several years earlier, but again the WHO's response was lukewarm. The Secretariat noted that the significant variations between regions made the elaboration of common, organization-wide and objective criteria more difficult than it might appear. The timetable set by the JIU was too tight and more consultation was needed.[99]

The 2012 JIU report noted that there are now 11 more country offices than when it last reported in 2001. It reiterated that the director-general and RDs, in consultation with member states, should agree on criteria for a minimum and robust country presence. The exercise first commissioned in 1998 should be completed. Criteria and procedures should also be developed on the opening and subsequent closing of the 137 sub-offices, subject to changing needs. The JIU noted that funds were spread very thinly among country offices, with 46 per cent of countries having a budget of $2 million or less. It also expressed concern that the number of staff in some country offices was so low as to cast doubt on how cost-effective their presence could be. A country presence might be desirable in as many countries as possible, but should only be maintained when there was a critical mass of properly qualified staff selected in relation to identified country needs. Otherwise, it would be more cost-effective to cover some countries from a neighbouring country office or from the regional office.

[94] Lucas, A. et al., 'Cooperation for Health Development: The World Health Organization's Support to Programmes at Country Level', September 1997, http://whqlibdoc. who.int/publications/0N02657577_V1_(ch1-ch2).pdf.http://whqlibdoc.who.int/publications/0N02657577_V1_(ch1-ch2).pdf; Cooperation for Health Development: WHO's Support to Programmes at Country Level. Summary, September 1997, http://www.norad.no/en/tools-and-publications/publications/publication?key=109668.
[95] *WHO Reform. WHO Country Offices. Report by the Director-General*, EB101/5, 4 December 1997, http://apps.who.int/gb/archive/pdf_files/EB101/pdfangl/ang5.pdf.
[96] *WHO Reform. WHO Country Offices: Criteria for Classifying Countries on the Basis of Need. Report by the Director-General*. EB102/2, 27 April 1998, http://apps.who.int/gb/archive/pdf_files/EB102/ee2.pdf.
[97] *Working in and with Countries. Report by the Director-General*, EB105/7, 15 December 1999, http://apps.who.int/gb/archive/pdf_files/EB105/ee7.pdf.
[98] 'Review of Management and Administration in the World Health Organization'.
[99] Reports of the Joint Inspection Unit, Review of Management and Administration in the World Health Organization, EB109/30,17 December 2001, http://apps.who.int/gb/archive/pdf_files/EB109/eeb10930.pdf.

Finally, the 2013 evaluation reiterated exactly the same point:

> WHO offices tend to vary widely in size and capacity, but only rarely in relation to a country's actual needs. What was already pointed out in a 1997 study of WHO's support to country level remains valid today. The [GPW] does not describe how WHO's future structure will match the core services it delivers in varying country settings, i.e. norm-setting, implementation, technical support, policy advice and advocacy. This is particularly important as Member States are going through wide-ranging economic, demographic and epidemiological changes that demand more resilient health systems and differentiated services. The changing Member States needs will require staff to have more than scientific skills, e.g. economics, diplomatic and strategy-making. While re-profiling has happened in certain countries (e.g. Thailand, India), it has not been done at an organisation-wide level. The GPW does not address this important dimension.[100]

Working group analysis

Our own analysis, based on WHO data, suggests that there remains great scope for considering the deployment of staff within the WHO, particularly at country level. We reclassified WHO country staffing according to the World Bank classification of countries by income level.

Table 1: Distribution of country staff by income group

Country income group	Number of countries	Number of staff	% of staff	Staff/ country
Low	35	1,445	42.5	41
Lower-middle	51	1,294	38.1	25
Upper-middle	46	586	17.2	13
High	16	75	2.2	5
All country offices	148	3,400	100.0	23

Sources: WHO Reform. Programmes and Priority Setting: Summary Information on the Distribution of Financial and Human Resources to Each Level and Cluster. EB130/5 Add.2, 13 January 2012, http://apps.who.int/gb/ebwha/pdf_files/EB130/B130_5Add2-en.pdf; Country and Lending Groups, World Bank, http://data.worldbank.org/about/country-classifications/country-and-lending-groups.

Table 1 indicates that while less than half of country staff are in the 35 low-income countries, more than 80 per cent are in low- and lower-middle-income countries. But the number of staff in each country varies widely – from one in each of several countries to 347 in Nigeria. As demonstrated in Annex 2, Table A1, larger offices are concentrated in low- and lower-middle-income countries, but there are sizeable offices in several upper-middle- and high-income countries – e.g. 102 in Angola, 45 in China, 44 in Fiji (a sub-regional office), 37 in Iraq, 29 in Thailand, 26 in South Africa, 24 in Russia and 23 in Iran.

At the same time, there are 60 countries each with fewer than 10 staff (see Annex 2, Table A2), concentrated in the upper-middle- and high-income groups. Of these, 23 offices are in PAHO countries where the actual staff complement is very much higher. In total, PAHO has a complement of 822 staff, of whom 366 are located outside the Washington headquarters. By contrast, WHO data record a PAHO headquarters headcount of 213, and country office staff numbering 100.

In many countries the nature of the support needed from the WHO was not to be measured by the number of projects, the funds transferred or the number of staff, but rather by the ability of the WHO to provide strategic advice. Often, the staffing of country offices was inappropriate to this kind of role.

The working group noted that in many countries the nature of the support needed from the WHO was not to be measured by the number of projects, the funds transferred or the number of staff, but rather by the ability of the WHO to provide strategic advice. Often, the staffing of country offices, in terms of numbers and skill set, was inappropriate to this kind of role. Too often, country offices were used as a supplement to, or indeed a substitute for, work that should be undertaken by the ministry of health. Again too often, country offices, because they appear to be a free resource, were used by countries in that role, sometimes to the detriment of building up national capacity. Apart from the way in which human and budgetary resources are deployed, there is a very wide variation in the capacities and skill sets in country offices. These are not necessarily tailored to country needs. There are many reports of countries demanding of WHO representatives expertise that they do not possess. The particular interests and skills of country representatives will tend to determine the nature of the assistance or advice offered – which may or may not be closely related to country needs, or to the WHO's stated priorities, or to what regional offices or headquarters might request them to do.

The location of country offices either within ministries of health or, if outside, in a close relationship with them can also distort country office perspectives so that they become 'demandeurs' from regional offices and headquarters on behalf of countries, rather than a source of independent advice and expertise. Sometimes they may also be at loggerheads with regional offices or headquarters, or find themselves

---

[100] Second Stage Evaluation on WHO Reform.

bypassed by the latter, for good or bad reasons. The closeness to the ministry of health can also be a handicap in dealing with other ministries with an influence on health, important in the context of the newer agendas on the social determinants of health and trade-related issues. Nor are country representatives sure exactly what they are – ambassadors of the WHO acting principally as diplomats, a technical assistance agency or a supplement to the ministry of health.

The working group felt that a different model was required for most country offices – i.e. fewer people, but more appropriately and highly skilled in response to country needs. At one extreme, one member said that the WHO could do its current work with just 2,000 staff. A member from a developing country explained it thus:

> Now what [my country] needs from WHO is policy support. I mean that [we] need WHO's input on policy advice. This need for support is increasing, not decreasing. What is decreasing is the [need for] support to specific projects. And up to now WHO's country office has spent a lot of time on the management of small but fragmented projects. They have a lot of staff working on that. But I don't think that's the role of WHO that is needed any more [We] need WHO's advice, support, for example in terms of health reform. How to improve universal access, how to reform the public hospital, and WHO can bring the international experience, negative or positive, to stimulate policy dialogue.

Another noted:

> What we expect from the WR [WHO Representatives] is [to] provide technical guidance, provide your social capital and intellectual capital. But because the WR office has been used to managing small projects it has become like a big boss giving us small money here and there. They don't know how to do this new function and they have difficulties. This is a big challenge […] but […] it hasn't been mentioned in most WHO discussions.

The working group considered that the WHO should focus on its role as a provider of global public goods that no other body had the credibility or legitimacy to provide. This should be at the core of its work. However, this did not mean that the WHO should not provide supportive functions to countries: this was very important. But the supportive role should be focused on helping countries to build capacity for, and implement, activities that flow from its core functions. These are topics related to its normative work in which the WHO itself is, in principle, the best provider of technical support – e.g. in helping countries to implement new treatment guidelines recommended by the WHO, in providing strategic advice on health system development, emergency response or IHR implementation.

Conclusions and proposals

The WHO's unique regional structure is deeply embedded in its history and political dynamics. While there is a widespread recognition that its decentralized structure carries significant costs and inefficiencies, which are manifested in different ways, there is also a pervasive resignation about the possibility of effecting any significant change in the current model.

The working group discussed, but did not agree on, two alternative proposals – a unitary model and a decentralized model.

Recommendation 7: The WHO should consider two alternative proposals for restructuring its regional offices:

- *Unitary:* The WHO should be like other UN organizations, where the need for regional (and country) offices is determined by what makes sense in terms of achieving organizational objectives. Elected regional directors should be phased out in order to allow structural changes to take place.

- *Decentralized:* The WHO should apply the PAHO model to the other regional offices; and the assessed contribution should be provided to regional offices directly by regional member states, rather than redistributed by HQ, Geneva. This would involve accepting a decentralized model in the WHO – or even the complete autonomy of regional offices, or their absorption by other regional organizations.

The staffing of country offices, the activities and skill sets required, what their essential purpose is, and how they should be distributed in the light of varying and evolving country needs have long been debated within the WHO. But, like the regional offices, and for many of the same reasons, there have always been reasons for not pursuing these issues with any vigour.

Recommendation 8: A comprehensive and independent review – of the kind that has been suggested since 1997 – is overdue to examine how the staffing of country offices should be matched to the needs of host countries, in particular with a view to translating WHO recommendations into practice.

5. Financing of the WHO

Introduction

The current concern about the preponderance of voluntary contributions in WHO financing often seems to imply a 'golden age' in which WHO activities were fully funded by assessed contributions. In fact, assessed contributions in the early years of the WHO generally amounted to between one-half and two-thirds of the total budget. From the beginning, moreover, there were prolonged arguments in the governing bodies about restraining assessed contributions. As early as 1949 the governing bodies 'recognized that, even to begin to meet the vast health needs of the world, considerable supplementary resources over and above the WHO regular budget would be required'.[101]

From 1951 onwards the WHO became the beneficiary of allocations from the Expanded Programme of Technical Assistance and the Special Fund, programmes set up by the UN to fund in particular the programmes of UN specialized agencies such as the WHO. In essence, these were voluntary contributions provided by major donor countries but allocated by a UN Technical Assistance Board or by the Special Fund. In 1951 just over 50 per cent of the WHO budget was financed by assessed contributions. By 1967, even with assessed contributions rising rapidly as the WHO's membership expanded, they still financed only two-thirds of WHO expenditure. Assessed contributions rose from $4.1 million in 1950 to $47.8 million in 1967. In the same period, the WHO's total income rose from $6.3 million to $72.2 million.[102]

> **For all the talk of financial crisis, the WHO's total revenues in 2012/13 at $4.9 billion were still the highest ever.**

Steps were therefore taken to raise voluntary contributions on top of those available from the UN programmes. In 1955 the WHA established the Malaria Eradication Special Account.[103] Then, in 1960 it established the Voluntary Fund for Health Promotion, which consolidated all the existing special accounts established for voluntary contributions. By 1996/97 assessed contributions still amounted, at $839 million, to more than 44 per cent of total income. It was only then that there began a precipitate decline in the share of assessed contributions, largely as a result of the enlarged inflow of voluntary contributions that occurred under Gro Harlem Brundtland as director-general. Thus the assessed share fell to 39 per cent in 1998/99, to 31 per cent in 2000/01, to less than 30 per cent in 2002/03 and to 21.5 per cent in 2012/13.[104]

Assessed and voluntary contributions

The most striking feature of the last 12 years has been the increase in voluntary contributions by member states (up by 138 per cent) and notably by non-member states (up by 258 per cent). In the same period, while voluntary contributions overall rose by 183 per cent, assessed contributions rose by only 13 per cent, and the WHO's total income from contributions rose by about 114 per cent. Global inflation, abstracting from exchange rate changes which may have adversely affected the WHO, was of the order of 25%, so the WHO's total income actually rose strongly in real terms. For all the talk of financial crisis, the WHO's total revenues in 2012/13 at $4.9 billion were still the highest ever.

Table 2: Assessed and voluntary contributions in 2000/01 and 2012/13 ($ million)

Country/ agency	Assessed contributions		Voluntary contributions		Total contributions	
	2000/01	*2012/13*	*2000/01*	*2012/13*	*2000/01*	*2012/13*
USA	216.2	219.8	147.9	394.7	364.1	614.5
Gates Foundation			11.0	567.7	11.0	567.7
United Kingdom	41.5	61.3	190.1	386.2	231.6	447.5
Canada	22.1	29.8	30.3	217.0	52.4	246.8
GAVI				222.9		222.9
Japan	169.4	116.4	17.9	33.0	187.3	149.4
Australia	12.1	18.0	19.0	127.2	31.1	145.2
Germany	80.9	74.5	6.7	70.2	87.6	144.7
Norway	5.0	8.1	48.1	121.5	53.1	129.6
European Commission			8.1	105.6	8.1	105.6
UNCERF				105.0		105.0
France	55.4	61.8	4.3	22.3	59.7	84.1
UNDP			0.6	81.1	0.6	81.1
Rotary International			61.8	79.6	61.8	79.6
Netherlands	13.3	17.2	169.1	48.0	182.4	65.2
Pakistan	0.5	0.8	0.0	52.2	0.5	53.0
Sweden	8.8	9.9	20.0	42.7	28.8	52.6
Top 11 member states	625.2	617.6	653.4	1,515.0	1,278.6	2,132.6
Total member states	842.7	949.2	758.0	1,807.9	1,600.7	2,757.1
% of total (top 11)	74.1	65.0	86.2	83.7	79.9	77.3
Total non-members			463.8	1,661.4	463.8	1,661.4
Total	842.7	949.2	1,221.8	3,469.3	2,064.5	4,418.5

Source: WHO Finance Reports.

---

[101] WHO, *The First Ten Years of the World Health Organization*; and *The Second Ten Years of the World Health* Organization, 1958–1967; http://whqlibdoc.who.int/publications/a38153.pdf.

[102] Ibid.

[103] World Health Organization, Resolution WHA8.30, May 1955, http://whqlibdoc.who.int/wha_eb_handbooks/9241652063_Vol1_(part1-2).pdf.

[104] Figures from successive Financial Report and Audited Financial Statements submitted to the WHA.

Table 2 shows that member-state funding is highly skewed. The top 11 countries account for more than three-quarters of this funding, particularly in the case of voluntary contributions, although rather less so in the case of assessed contributions. The table also shows, for comparison, the top voluntary contributors to the WHO. As noted above, the most notable feature is the Bill & Melinda Gates Foundation, which by 2012/13 had become the largest single voluntary contributor to the WHO and the second largest contributor in total after the United States. In fact in 2013 the Foundation was the largest single contributor to the WHO ($301.3 million against the United States' assessed and voluntary contribution of $289.6 million). It should be noted that the private sector contributed in 2012/13 only about 1% of total contributions, in the form of a large number of mainly small amounts from many different companies (Figure 4).

Figure 4: Voluntary contributions in 2012/13 by source (%)

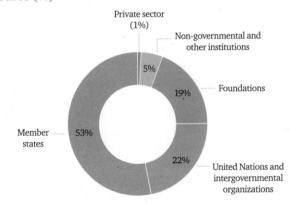

Source: Financial Report and Audited Financial Statements for the year ended 31 December 2013, A67/43.

The allocation of funds

In theory, the WHA only approves the operations of the WHO that are funded by assessed contributions (and some other income such as interest). By contrast, activities funded by voluntary contributions are determined in negotiations between the WHO secretariat and the funder. That is why the centre point of the current reform programme in the WHO is an experiment whereby the WHA approves the WHO's total budget and then the WHO attempts, through a financing dialogue with funders, to align the allocations of funders with the priorities identified in the WHA-approved budget.

A major concern in the reform programme has been the fact that the great majority of voluntary contributions are earmarked for particular activities agreed with the donor, and

the resulting inability of the WHO to respond meaningfully to priorities agreed by member states in the WHA (see Chapter 3, concerning unfunded commitments agreed to by the WHA). In the last few years some countries have agreed to include an element of highly or moderately flexible funding in their voluntary contributions (the core voluntary contributions account) to offset to some extent the impact of the relative decline in assessed contributions as a proportion of the budget. Based on hoped-for progress in the reform process, the 2012/13 programme budget foresaw that, out of total projected voluntary contributions of just over $3 billion, $400 million would be in the form of 'highly flexible' funding and $400 million in the form of 'medium flexible' funding. However, in 2012/13 the former category actually amounted to $231 million and the latter to just $33 million, compared with figures in 2010/11 of $235 million and $14 million respectively. While overall voluntary contributions in 2012/13 exceeded the amounts foreseen in the programme budget by about $450 million – funds that will be carried over for use in the succeeding biennium – the trend was therefore exactly the opposite of what was intended in the reform programme. As compared with the projected share of 'flexible funding' of 27 per cent for voluntary contributions, the out-turn was only 7.6 per cent. Overall in 2012/13, 72.5 per cent of the WHO's funding for the programme budget was in the form of earmarked contributions. Although the financing dialogue with donors is in its early days, the willingness of member states and other contributors to increase funding flexibility in practice has yet to be demonstrated.[105]

The situation is complicated because assessed contributions from member states typically come from ministries of health or sometimes ministries of foreign affairs, while voluntary contributions typically come from development and other ministries or agencies. Assessed contributions come as one transaction per country, while voluntary contributions come in a bewildering variety of separate transactions from different agencies within the donor country, or from non-state donors, and from different arms of the same agency – each requiring a separate memorandum of understanding.

The figures for the top contributors in 2012 (Table 3) confirm this complexity. The third column illustrates the number of different components (i.e. grants or separate sub-components of grants) that are associated with each contributor. In total, the WHO accounted for voluntary contributions on 1,738 separate lines in 2012, of which the top 10 donors are responsible for 683 (and for 69 per cent of total voluntary contributions). The United States has by far the largest number of separate projects with the WHO and includes funding from many US government bodies (such as the National Institutes of Health, USAID and the CDC).

[105] Financial Report and Audited Financial Statements for the year ended 31 December 2013, A67/43, 17 April 2014, http://apps.who.int/gb/ebwha/pdf_files/WHA67/A67_43-en.pdf.

Table 3: Top 10 voluntary contributors in 2012 ($ million)

Contributor	Contribution	No. of awards
Gates Foundation	271.2	46
United States	237.5	309
United Kingdom	131.7	31
Canada	99.6	21
GAVI	92.6	22
Australia	67.9	28
European Commission	65.7	94
Norway	57.8	32
UNCERF	54.9	83
Rotary International	42.9	17
Total	1,122.0	683

Source: WHO Finance Reports.

Apart from the transactions costs associated with voluntary contributions, the division between the principal providers of assessed and voluntary contributions accentuates a difference in perspective between those who sit in the WHO's governance bodies from ministries of health, and those who provide the bulk of voluntary funding – mainly from development agencies, which are not generally represented in those bodies. To this latter group, the WHO has something of the appearance of a free delivery vehicle for health-sector projects. Whatever its perceived faults and inefficiencies, it provides a ready-made infrastructure with worldwide coverage without the need to set up a separate organization for such projects.

The WHO's finances are for the most part opaque ... it is very difficult to know exactly where resources are allocated – for what purpose, and for what result.

The WHO's finances are for the most part opaque. Aggregate figures are presented to governing bodies, and auditors endorse the financial statements, but it is very difficult to know exactly where resources are allocated – for what purpose, and for what result. Detail not available at the global level might be provided by the regional offices, but with one or two exceptions the detail provided publicly by regional offices is very limited. Whereas WHO headquarters meticulously publishes every document presented to the EB, its subcommittee the Programme Budget and Administration Committee (PBAC), and the WHA, the information provided

by regional offices is patchy – particularly as regards the budgetary items. To take one example, the information provided on the 2012 SEARO regional committee contains a list of the documents considered but not the documents themselves.[106] The Administration and Finance page of the SEARO website contains no budgetary information at all.[107] For AFRO, the web page on Resources and Planning provides minimal information.[108] By contrast, EURO provides access to documentation in a similar way to WHO headquarters on governance.[109] PAHO provides comprehensive information via a Subcommittee on Program, Budget and Administration.[110]

This reinforces the views of the 2012 JIU report on the quality of regional governance, noted above. The reality is that where the member states of regions are not providing resources directly to support regional offices, the incentives for better oversight by member states are strictly limited. The emphasis necessarily tends to be on how much is being distributed from Geneva, not the consideration of whether money is being spent effectively or how it could be better allocated. For example, in 2013 the SEARO regional committee approved the 2014/15 programme budget, while also asking the RD to take up with the director-general the 11.5 per cent cut that it had received in its budget.[111] Thus, other than in the case of PAHO, where member states do contribute the majority of the budget directly, it is not surprising that the level of oversight of finance and management issues is deficient.

Funding of the three WHO levels

None of the WHO's budgetary documents adequately explain the basis on which spending is allocated between countries, regions and headquarters. For instance, it is known that spending by regional offices or headquarters may be country-specific, but will not necessarily be recorded in country office budgets. Similarly, since a primary purpose of regional offices must be to support countries, rather than work specifically of a regional nature, the concept of regional spending not devoted to countries, or a group of countries, is somewhat hard to conceptualize.

In recent years a 30/70 headquarters/regional split has been an implicit, if not explicit, objective of policy. It is essentially a politically determined rather than an evidence-based policy. This was made clear when JW Lee was campaigning to become director-general in 2003. He suggested to the EB that:

---

[106] http://www.searo.who.int/about/governing_bodies/regional_committee/65/rc65_lod.pdf.
[107] http://www.searo.who.int/about/administration_structure/administration_finance/en/index.html.
[108] http://www.afro.who.int/en/who-in-the-african-region/resources-and-planning.html.
[109] http://www.euro.who.int/en/who-we-are/governance/regional-committee-for-europe/sixty-second-session/documentation/working-documents.
[110] Subcommittee on Program, Budget and Administration, http://www.paho.org/hq/index.php?option=com_content&view=article&id=684&Itemid=711&lang=en.
[111] Proposed Programme Budget 2014–2015, SEA/RC66/R3, 13 September 2013, http://www.searo.who.int/mediacentre/events/governance/rc/66/r3.pdf?ua=1.

I will devote more of WHO's resources to the countries and regions where they can have the most direct impact. Today, the numbers of staff, long-term and short-term, at HQ are increasing steadily. In the 2004 and 2005 budget, 36% of the total are allocated to HQ. I will shift this HQ proportion to 25% by 2005 and 20% by 2008. Shifting the HQ budget to the regions and countries will stop and reverse the trend of ever increasing number of HQ staff.[112]

This proved wildly overambitious, but may have helped him in his election campaign.

Tables 4 and 5 indicate that meeting the 30/70 target has proved elusive. While the budget for 2010/11 was close to the 30 per cent target for headquarters, the out-turn figures show that headquarters actually received more than 42 per cent of funding. The headquarters' share of actual funding was higher in 2010/11 than in 2000/01. However, the out-turn in 2012/13, with headquarters receiving 31.7 per cent of funding, was the closest ever reached in a biennium, and in 2013 alone the 30 per cent target

Table 4: Resource allocation by office ($ million)

	AFRO	AMRO	EMRO	EURO	SEARO	WPRO	HQ	Total
2000/01 out-turn	673.4	90.0	171.9	122.7	187.0	118.9	812.2	2,176.1
%	30.9	4.1	7.9	5.6	8.6	5.5	37.3	100.0
2010/11 out-turn	1,041.4	158.0	448.8	203.5	337.1	267.9	1,834.3	4,320.4
%	24.1	3.7	10.4	4.7	7.8	6.2	42.5	100.0
2012/13 budget	1,093.1	173.1	553.5	213.3	384.2	245.7	1,296.0	3,959.0
%	27.6	4.4	14.0	5.4	9.7	6.2	32.7	100.0
2012/13 out-turn	1,138.0	131.2	630.0	203.9	349.9	263.2	1,259.3	3,975.6
%	28.6	3.3	15.8	5.1	8.8	6.6	31.7	100.0
2014/15 budget	1,112.0	176.0	560.0	230.0	340.0	270.0	1,281.0	3,977.0
%	28.0	4.4	14.1	5.8	8.5	6.8	32.2	100.0

Sources: Programme Budgets, Financial Reports and Accounts.

Table 5: Country and regional financing ($ million)

	Countries	Regions	Countries/regions	Headquarters	Total
2000/01 out-turn	663.1	700.8	1,363.9	812.2	2,176.1
%	30.5	32.2	62.7	37.3	100.0
2004/05 out-turn	1,061.4	819.0	1,880.4	1,151.6	3,032.0
%	35.0	27.0	62.0	38.0	100.0
2008/09 budget	1,811.6	1,240.0	3,051.6	1,175.9	4,227.5
%	42.9	29.3	72.2	27.8	100.0
2008/09 out-turn			2,453.7	1,412.1	3,865.8
%			63.5	36.5	100.0
2010/11 budget	2,043.7	1,107.0	3,150.7	1,389.2	4,539.9
%	45.0	24.4	69.4	30.5	100.0
2010/11 out-turn			2,486.1	1,834.3	4,320.4
%			57.5	42.5	100.0
2012/13 budget			2,663.0	1,296.0	3,959.0
%			67.3	32.7	100.0
2012/13 out-turn			2,716.3	1,259.3	3,975.6
%			68.3	31.7	100.0
2014/15 budget	1,890.1	800.9	2,691.0	1,286.2	3,977.2
%	47.5	20.1	67.7	32.3	100.0

Sources: Programme Budgets, Financial Reports and Accounts.

---

[112] Presentation to the Executive Board, 27 January 2003, http://www.who.int/dg/lee/speeches/2003/en/.

was exactly reached. In respect of spending in countries, comparisons are hampered because the last set of out-turn figures that recorded country spending separately from regional spending was in 2004/05. In that biennium 41.3 per cent of expenditure was budgeted for countries, but actual expenditure turned out to be only 35 per cent. Since the headquarters (and regional office) share has, until 2012/13, proved so resistant to decline, it is open to question whether the 47.5 per cent budgeted for countries in 2014/15 will be reached.

Core functions and assured funding

The WHO's existence in its current form depends on mainly earmarked voluntary contributions. The fact is that these now meet 75–80 per cent of all WHO costs, and more than 60 per cent of staff costs. Put another way, the WHO's total staff costs, although down to $1.8 billion in 2012/13 from $1.96 billion in 2010/11, are still nearly double the assessed contribution (about $950 million). Similarly, the total cost of operations at headquarters in Geneva, although significantly reduced in 2012/13, is one-third more than the assessed contribution, and the cost of the Africa regional and country offices alone is significantly more than the assessed contribution.

The WHO is funded in a number of ways by a multiplicity of governmental and non-governmental institutions to undertake a range of activities relevant to promoting global health. The question is whether these are the activities that it should be performing, and whether it is undertaking them in the most efficient ways.

It is often claimed, including in the recent study commissioned from PwC as part of the reform programme,[113] that the WHO has to subsidize from its regular budget the overheads imposed on it to administer programmes financed by voluntary contributions. This is difficult to square with the reality that voluntary contributions – as a result of their sheer volume – allow the WHO to be about four times the size it would be in their absence, and that many 'core' programmes (and their staff) only exist because of voluntary contributions. The following examples illustrate this:

- The Expert Committee on Specifications for Pharmaceutical Preparations was first established as the Expert Committee on Unification of Pharmacopoeias by the WHO Interim Commission in 1947. According to an official WHO history, whereas its activities were largely financed in the past by the regular budget (assessed contributions), in the last few years only about 10 per cent of funding has come from that source, and 90 per cent from different voluntary contributors.[114]

- The WHO's prequalification programme was established in 2001 and may be regarded as a critical contribution by the WHO to increasing access to medicines for priority diseases, harmonizing quality standards for generic manufacturers and transferring skills to developing countries.[115] But 85 per cent of its funding is provided by UNITAID, and 100 per cent from outside the WHO.[116]

- The WHO's past and present eradication campaigns for malaria, smallpox and now polio have been mainly financed by voluntary contributions.

It is not at all clear that the regular budget is in reality cross-subsidizing activities funded by voluntary contributions. This quite narrow technicality seems to be entirely secondary to the systemic questions raised by the preponderance of voluntary contributions in the WHO's funding. The fact is that without voluntary contributions the WHO would be able to do less of its 'core' work, however that might be defined. So it is a moot question which way the cross-subsidization goes.

WHO structure and cost-effectiveness

The reality is that the WHO is funded in a number of ways by a multiplicity of governmental and non-governmental institutions to undertake a range of activities relevant to promoting global health. The question is whether these are the activities that it should be performing, and whether it is undertaking them in the most efficient ways. The PwC cost study points out that the WHO's administrative and management (A&M) costs amount to 31–33 per cent of total WHO expenditure or about $1.3 billion per biennium, or 30 per cent if the costs of funding member state and external expert travel is excluded. Thus the WHO's A&M costs alone exceed the regular budget by over one-third.

[113] Administration and Management Cost Study, EBPBAC 18/3, 12 April 2013, http://apps.who.int/gb/pbac/pdf_files/Eighteenth/PBAC18_3-en.pdf.
[114] Expert Committee on Specifications for Pharmaceutical Preparations: Outcome of 44 Meetings, WHO, Geneva, 2011, http://apps.who.int/medicinedocs/documents/s18645en/s18645en.pdf.
[115] 't Hoen, E. et al., 'A Quiet Revolution in Global Public Health: The World Health Organization's Prequalification of Medicines Programme', *Journal of Public Health Policy* (2014), Vol. 35 (2): 137–61.
[116] Annual Report 2012, WHO Prequalification of Medicines Programme, WHO, Geneva, 2012, http://apps.who.int/prequal.

The study takes these A&M costs as a given, as implicitly does the internal reform programme. Neither questions whether these are too high, or considers ways in which they might be reduced. Rather, there is an acceptance that this is something that has to be lived with: the problem is how to get them funded through assessed or voluntary contributions and preferably in a more secure way.

However, the study does point to a number of reasons why the WHO's administrative cost structure could be considered to be so high:

- **Geographical footprint.** The WHO is one of the UN agencies with the broadest footprint in terms of regional and country offices. This includes presence in security-compromised areas and locations with poor infrastructure, which typically drives security and telecommunication costs up. As noted above, typically over 60 per cent of WHO expenditure is in country and regional offices, and about three-quarters of staff are employed in these.

- **Funding model.** The WHO's dual financing model and the types of donors have an impact on A&M costs. There are more than 200 voluntary contributors to the WHO, and, as noted above, the larger donors have multiple separate agreements with it. The study estimates that the A&M costs associated with voluntary contributions approach $500 million per biennium.

- **Governance.** The WHO has a complex governance model. The WHA, the EB and subcommittees, six regional committees and their subcommittees, six official languages, and travel costs for some member states make the WHO extremely expensive to run before the cost of any actual activities is taken into account. PwC estimates that the WHO basic running costs covering what used to be termed strategic objectives 12 and 13[117] constitute more than $800 million of total A&M costs of $1.3 billion per biennium.[118]

The key point made in this report is that it is quite possible that the costs of governance, and of the regional and country offices, could be significantly reduced without adversely affecting the WHO's effectiveness; or that by removing some the inefficiencies intrinsic to the existing three-tiered structure, as outlined above, its effectiveness could be enhanced.

Conclusion

The WHO has always been reliant on voluntary contributions, even from the early days, but in the last five years the share of these in its funding has exceeded 75 per cent. The WHO's problem is not inadequate income. Rather, it is the imbalance between what member states, through the governing bodies, and voluntary contributors (including member states), through separate agreements, ask the WHO to do, the means offered to achieve what is asked, and the WHO's capacity to use those means to best effect. Any programme of reform needs to undertake a serious review of the major cost centres – in particular administration and management, the cost of which is directly related to the WHO's extensive network of country and regional offices, and to the governance mechanisms associated with the WHO's unique regional structure. This needs to be done in the context of considering what functions the WHO should be undertaking and what can be done at least as well by others. This report argues that a comprehensive reform programme should concentrate on these structural issues concerning governance and cost-effectiveness, and that a WHO focused on its core tasks could do more good with less money. The WHO's member states have so far been unwilling to tackle these structural issues in the reform programme.

Recommendation 9: The WHO and its member states should examine how its effectiveness could be enhanced by reviewing – in conjunction with the other recommendations in this report – how the value added by its regional and country offices could be increased, and its administrative and management costs reduced.

Recommendations

1. The WHO's core functions should provide explicitly for its work in promoting and maintaining global health security.

2. The WHO should provide strategic technical assistance to countries in support of its mission as a provider of global public goods. It should not seek to undertake activities that could or should be done better by others – by the host government, with or without support from other agencies.

3. The WHO should undertake a review of the skills mix and expertise of its staff to ensure that it fits with its core functions and leadership priorities.

---

[117] SO 12: 'To provide leadership, strengthen governance and foster partnership and collaboration with countries, the United Nations system, and other stakeholders in order to fulfil the mandate of WHO in advancing the global health agenda as set out in the Eleventh General Programme of Work.' SO 13: 'To develop and sustain WHO as a flexible, learning organization, enabling it to carry out its mandate more efficiently and effectively.'
[118] Administration and Management Cost Study, EBPBAC 18/3,12 April 2013, http://apps.who.int/gb/pbac/pdf_files/Eighteenth/PBAC18_3-en.pdf.

4. The WHO should provide an internal separation between its technical departments and those dealing with governance and management by creating two posts of deputy director-general, with one to be responsible for each.

5. The WHO should allow the director-general a single, seven-year term, without the possibility of re-election.

6. The WHO should explore new avenues for collaboration with non-governmental actors that have a concrete and specific purpose.

7. The WHO should consider two alternative proposals for restructuring its regional offices:

- *Unitary*: The WHO should be like other UN organizations, where the need for regional (and country) offices is determined by what makes sense in terms of achieving organizational objectives. Elected regional directors should be phased out in order to allow structural changes to take place.

- *Decentralized*: The WHO should apply the PAHO model to the other regional offices; and the assessed contribution should be provided to regional offices direct by regional member states, rather than redistributed by HQ, Geneva. This would involve accepting a decentralized model – or even the complete autonomy of regional offices, or their absorption by other regional organizations.

8. A comprehensive and independent review – of the kind that has been suggested since 1997 – is overdue to examine how the staffing of country offices should be matched to the needs of host countries, in particular with a view to translating WHO recommendations into practice.

9. The WHO and its member states should examine how its effectiveness could be enhanced by reviewing, in conjunction with the other recommendations in this report, how the value added by its regional and country offices could be increased, and its administrative and management costs reduced.

Annex 1: Working Group Members

Name	Country	Affiliation
Working Group 1		
Working Group Members attending at least one meeting		
Viroj Tangcharoensathien	Thailand	Ministry of Public Health
José Roberto de Andrade Filho	Brazil	UN Mission, Geneva
Fran Baum	Australia	Flinders University/People's Health Movement
Sally Davies	United Kingdom	Department of Health
David Fidler	USA	Indiana University
Jane Halton	Australia	Department of Health and Ageing
Larry Gostin	USA	Georgetown University
Peilong Liu	China	Ministry of Health
Ann Marie Kimball/Stephen Landry	USA	Bill & Melinda Gates Foundation
Precious Matsoso	South Africa	Ministry of Health
Anne Mills	United Kingdom	London School of Hygiene and Tropical Medicine
Sigrun Møgedal	Norway	Norwegian Knowledge Centre
Anders Nordström	Sweden	Ministry of Foreign Affairs
Srinath Reddy	India	Public Health Foundation
Working Group Members who did not attend a meeting		
Tim Evans	Canada	World Bank
Tom Mboya	Kenya	Geneva UN Ambassador
Keizo Takemi	Japan	Japan Centre for International Exchange
Others who participated or presented		
K Churnrurtai	Thailand	Prince Mahidol University
Steven Hoffman	Canada	McMaster University
Monir Islam	Bangladesh	WHO/SEARO
Jon Lidén	Norway	Consultant
Anna Miyagi	Japan	Ministry of Foreign Affairs
Jadej Thammatach-Aree	Thailand	London School of Hygiene and Tropical Medicine

Annex 2: Country Office Staffing

Table A1: Larger WHO offices by income group

Office size	Low	Lower-middle	Upper-middle	High
10–24	Eritrea (24), Comoros (21), Togo (21), Gambia (20) Guinea-Bissau (14), Tajikistan (14)	Senegal (24), Mauritania (23), Swaziland (22), Philippines (21), Ukraine (20), Mongolia (18), Yemen, Rep (19), Lesotho (17), Timor-Leste (17), Uzbekistan (17), Bhutan (12), Egypt (12), Cape Verde (11), Samoa (10), São Tomé and Príncipe (10)	Iran (23), Namibia (19), Botswana (15), Maldives (15), Turkey (15), Serbia (14), Albania (13), Brazil (12)*, Azerbaijan (11), Libya (11)	Russian Federation (24), Equatorial Guinea (18)
25–49	Tanzania (46), Cambodia (45), Somalia (45), Sierra Leone (40), Niger (37), Liberia (35), Madagascar (34), Burkina Faso (32), Guinea (32), Central African Republic (29), Mozambique (29), Mali (28), Rwanda (27), Benin (26), Burundi (26), Malawi (26)	Côte d'Ivoire (37), Ghana (37), Lao PDR (36), Cameroon (31), Papua New Guinea (30), Zambia (30), Sri Lanka (27), West Bank and Gaza (27), Congo, Rep (26)	China (45), Fiji (44), Iraq (37), Thailand (29), South Africa (26)	
50–99	Afghanistan (79), Chad (64), Kenya (61), Myanmar (59), Nepal (57), Uganda (52), Bangladesh (50), Zimbabwe (50)	Indonesia (79), Sudan (69), Vietnam (65), Pakistan (62), India (51)		
Over 100	Ethiopia (153), Congo DR (150)	Nigeria (347)	Angola (102)	

*Brazil has 52 staff, including PAHO funding.
Sources: WHO Reform, Programmes and Priority Setting: Summary Information on the Distribution of Financial and Human Resources to Each Level and Cluster, EB130/5 Add.2, 13 January 2012, http://apps.who.int/gb/ebwha/pdf_files/EB130/B130_5Add2-en.pdf; Country and Lending Groups, World Bank, http://data.worldbank.org/about/country-classifications/country-and-lending-groups; PASB Staffing Statistics, CSP28/INF/4 (Eng.), 2 July 2012, http://www.paho.org/hq/index.php?option=com_content&view=article&id=7022&Itemid=39541&lang=en.

Table A2: Smaller WHO offices by income group*

Office size	Low	Lower-middle	Upper-middle	High
1		Paraguay (8)	Suriname (3)	Bahamas (3), Estonia, Korea, Rep, Uruguay (14)
2		Nicaragua (13)	Argentina (13), Montenegro, Romania, Venezuela (10)	Lithuania, Chile (7), Croatia, Slovakia, Slovenia
3	Haiti (12)	Kiribati	Hungary, Bulgaria, Costa Rica (12), Turkmenistan	Czech Republic
4		El Salvador (10), Guyana (7), Honduras (11)	Panama (15), Tonga	Poland, Trinidad and Tobago (20)
5		Bolivia (14), Guatemala (17), Syrian Arab Republic	Belarus, Colombia (14), Jamaica (14)	
6		Vanuatu	Dominican Republic (11), Ecuador (12), Mexico (15), Seychelles, Tunisia	Saudi Arabia
7		Armenia, Georgia	Bosnia and Herzegovina, Kazakhstan, Macedonia, Peru (25)	
8	Korea, Dem Rep, Kyrgyz Republic	Djibouti, Morocco	Lebanon, Malaysia, Mauritius	
9		Moldova, Solomon Islands	Algeria, Jordan	

*Figures in parentheses indicate staffing including PAHO funding.
Sources: As Table A1.

The Centre on Global Health Security Working Group Papers

Working Group on Financing

Paper 1: Development Assistance for Health: Critiques and Proposals for Change
Suerie Moon and Oluwatosin Omole
April 2013
ISBN 978 1 86203 285 9
http://www.chathamhouse.org/publications/papers/
view/190951

Paper 2: Raising and Spending Domestic Money for Health
Riku Elovainio and David B. Evans
May 2013
ISBN 978 1 86203 286 6
http://www.chathamhouse.org/publications/papers/
view/191335

Paper 3: Development Assistance for Health: Quantitative Allocation Criteria and Contribution Norms
Trygve Ottersen, Aparna Kamath, Suerie Moon, John-Arne Røttingen
February 2014
ISBN 978 1 78413 001 5
http://www.chathamhouse.org/publications/papers/
view/197643

Paper 4: Financing Global Health Through a Global Fund for Health?
Gorik Ooms and Rachel Hammonds
February 2014
ISBN 978 1 78413 002 2
http://www.chathamhouse.org/publications/papers/
view/197444

Paper 5: Fiscal Space for Domestic Funding of Health and Other Social Services
Di McIntyre and Filip Meheus
March 2014
ISBN 978 1 78413 005 3
http://www.chathamhouse.org/publications/papers/
view/198263

Working Group on Governance

Paper 1: The Role of the World Health Organization in the International System
Charles Clift
February 2013
ISBN 978 1 86203 281 1
http://www.chathamhouse.org/publications/papers/
view/189351

Paper 2: The Grand Decade for Global Health: 1998–2008
Jon Lidén
April 2013
ISBN 978 1 86203 282 8
http://www.chathamhouse.org/publications/papers/
view/190715

Paper 3: The World Health Organization in the South East Asia Region: Decision-maker Perceptions
Devaki Nambiar, with Preety Rajbangshi and Kaveri Mayra
April 2014
ISBN 978 1 78413 006 0
http://www.chathamhouse.org/publications/papers/
view/199260

Working Groups on Antimicrobial Resistance

Paper 1: New Business Models for Sustainable Antibiotics
Kevin Outterson
February 2014
ISBN 978 1 74813 003 9
http://www.chathamhouse.org/publications/papers/
view/197446